For permissions requests or inquiries,
please contact:

Camille Eliott
868-713-8869

ISBN: 9798395482914

Printed and bound by Amazon

NOSOCOMIAL INFECTIONS IN TRINIDAD AND TOBAGO

A Thesis
Submitted in Fulfillment of the Requirement for the Degree of Master
of Philosophy in Medical Microbiology

of
The University of the West Indies

by
Camille Elliott
2023

Department of Para-Clinical Science
Faculty of Medical Science
St. Augustine Campus

ABSTRACT

Nosocomial Infections in Trinidad and Tobago

Camille Elliott

Infections acquired in health care settings are major causes of death and increased morbidity among hospitalized patients. The most frequent nosocomial infections are infections of surgical wounds, urinary tract and blood stream. Infection rates are higher among patients who are with increased risk factors such as extremes of age, underlying disease or long term stay in hospital. There is limited data available on the epidemiology of nosocomial infections in Trinidad and Tobago. The objectives of this research were to investigate the: frequency of all types of nosocomial infections especially nosocomial urinary tract infections, frequency of multiple drug resistance among bacterial organisms associated with nosocomial infections, infection control measures practiced at some hospitals in Trinidad and Tobago and cost of such nosocomial infections in terms of morbidity and mortality.

In this study, a prospective cross sectional study design was applied. Standard data form was used to obtain demographic and clinical information of all patients assessed as having hospital acquired infections. The nosocomial pathogens where possible were retrieved from the microbiology laboratory. These were further identified using conventional laboratory methods.

A breakdown of the research findings revealed that: 450 in patients were associated with nosocomial infections with thirty (30) mortalities during the twelve (12) month study (June 2013 to May 2014) at the three (3) Regional hospitals. The incidence was 5.8% and the nosocomial rate was 3.6 per 1000, (450/126,668). The highest nosocomial rate of 30.1% was observed in the Intensive Care Unit (82/272 admissions). Skin and Soft Tissue Nosocomial Infections, 168 (37.3%) was the most frequent type of nosocomial infections. *Staphylococcus spp,* (193/859)*Pseudomonas aeroginosa ssp* (109/859), *Acinetobacter* (101/859) and *Klebsiella spp.* (100/859) were the most frequently occurring nosocomial pathogens.

Consistency in practicing good infection management is vital in reducing the nosocomial rates and incidences at the research sites. Of the 450 cases recovered from all three research sites during the research period special attention should be given to the ICU ward, as the nosocomial rate (82/272 admissions), was the highest. Surgical wards too should be given key focus; as Surgical wards (152/450) accounted for having the highest frequency of nosocomial infections.

Keywords: Cross sectional study; incidence; mortalities; Nosocomial Infections – (NI's); susceptibility patterns; Trinidad and Tobago and West Indies.

ACKNOWLEDGEMENTS

This thesis would have remained a dream had it not been for God's sustaining grace that equipped me with the determination needed, coupled with the continual effective fervent prayers and support from my family and love-ones. It is with immense gratitude that I acknowledge the: support and help of advisory committee members, respective regional health authority members, respective nurses, doctors, laboratory personnel's at research sites for the roles they played in ensuring the success of my research. I am also indebted to my fellow colleagues for the encouragement and motivation they have demonstrated.

I would like to express my deepest gratitude to my advisor, Professor Patrick E. Akpaka, for his excellent guidance and motivating drive which allowed me to demonstrate great enthusiasm to conduct my research and Dr. Vaillant in helping me in the publication stages of my thesis. I would like to thank Mr. Frank, Dr. Legal and Dr. Randy Seepersad who devoted their time to make available the following practical experience with SPSS software beyond the text-books. I would also like to extend appreciation to my father and other sponsors for financially supporting me being self-sponsored with my graduate research and my mother, my coach, for all the mentorship, motivation and drive she gave me.

I consider it a great honor to work along with Dr. Ana Navas and Mr. John at the San Fernando General Hospital Laboratory. I am very appreciative of their guidance in my graduate research for the past several months and helping me to develop my practical background in the laboratories. I would like to thank Mr. Blake and Dr. Saleh, who as good colleagues were always willing to help and give their best suggestions while doing the graduate research and writing up the publications. It would have been a lonely research without them and the motivation from my other beloved colleagues as well.

Many thanks to Ms. Nicole, Ms. Patrina, Ms. Angie and other laboratory staff personnels from the laboratories governed by Dr. Swanston, Dr. Wesley Greaves and Dr. Manjunath from the Mt. Hope, San Fernando and Port of Spain General Hospital laboratories for facilitating me in using their laboratories and collecting samples of interest needed and storing and processing in their respective laboratories while conducting my research. My research would not have been possible without their help. I would also like to thank my only elder sister, Christine Elliott. She has always been supporting me and encouraging me with her best wishes.

Finally, I would like to thank my church family and God. They were always there cheering me up and stood by my side through the good and bad moments.

DEDICATION

I dedicate my thesis work to my grand-father, the late Mr. Egbert Bean who was an activist for educational right amongst other rights in his district. A special feeling of gratitude to him, my loving parents Mrs. Angella Elliott, an educator, registered teacher and librarian and Mr. Alexander Elliott, a successful businessman and cop, family and friends whose words of encouragement and push for tenacity rang in my ears and have taught me from their experiences; how from very humbled background to achieve honestly with integrity and humility in becoming a true successor. My sister, Christine Elliott, has never left my side and is very special.

I also dedicate this thesis book to my many friends and church family who have supported me throughout the process. I will always appreciate all they have done; especially Auntie Claris Allen affectionately called, for helping me develop my inner strength, Auntie Heather Bean for the many moments of re-assurance and Pastor Everton Mapp for helping me to master the leader dots.

I dedicate this work and give special thanks to Jesus Christ for being there for me throughout the entire Masters of Philosophy in Medical Microbiology (MPhil Med MicroB) Program. Jesus, you have been my best cheer-leader.

TABLE OF CONTENTS

CHAPTER TWO

2.0 LITERATURE REVIEW

CHAPTER THREE

3.0 METHODOLOGY

LIST OF FIGURES

LIST OF TABLES

LIST OF ACRONYMNS

ADD	....	Agar Disk Diffusion
AK	....	Amikacin
AMC	....	Amoxicillin/Clavulanic acid
AML	....	Amoxillin
AMP	....	Ampicillin
ATM	....	Aztreonam
ATP	....	Adenosine triphosphate
BSI	....	Blood Stream Infection
CAZ	....	Ceftazidime
CDC	....	Centers for Disease Control and Prevention
CEF	....	Cefaclor
CIP	....	Ciprofloxacin
CLSI	....	Clinical and Laboratory Standards Institute
CNSI	....	Central Nervous System Infection
CT	....	Colistin Sulfate
CXM	....	Cefuroxime
DA	....	Clindamycin
ERIC	....	Enterobacterial Repetitive Intergenic Consensus
ETP	....	Ertapenem
EWMSC	....	Eric Williams Medical Sciences Complex

F	……………..	Nitrofurantoin
FEP	…………….	Cefepime
GN	…………….	Gentamicin
HAI	…………….	Hospital Acquired Infection
ICU	…………….	Intensive Care Unit
IMP	…………….	Imipenem
LEV	…………….	Levofloxacin
LZD	……………..	Linezolid
MDRO	…………….	Multi-Drug Resistant Organism
MEM	…………….	Meropenem
MIC	…………….	Minimum Inhibitory Concentration
NI	…………….	Nosocomial Infection
NNIS	…………….	National Nosocomial Infections Surveillance
NOR	…………….	Norfloxacin
PICU	……………..	Pediatric Intensive Care Unit
PIP	…………….	Piperacillin
POSGH	…………….	Port of Spain General Hospital
RHA	…………….	Regional Health Authority
RTI	…………….	Respiratory Tract Infection

SFGH	....	San Fernando General Hospital
SSTI	....	Skin and Soft Tissue Infection
SXT	....	Trimethoprine/Sulphamethazole
TE	....	Tetracycline
TGC	....	Tigercycline
TOB	....	Tobramycin
TZP	....	Piperacillin/Tazobactam
UTI	....	Urinary Tract Infection
WHO	....	World Health Organization

CHAPTER 1

1.0 Introduction

1.1 Epidemiology of Nosocomial Infection

In spite of increasing efforts to reduce its incidence worldwide, nosocomial infections (NI) otherwise referred to as hospital acquired infections (HAI), continue to be an ever growing threat to the commitment of improving quality of care provided to in patients in hospitals. Hospital acquired infections are major reasons for disease and deaths in several countries including the United States of America, Europe, Benin, Trinidad and Tobago and Jamaica. According to the National Nosocomial Infections Surveillance system, NNIS [50]; available report states that within the period of 1975 and 1995, the nosocomial rates increased by 36% from 7.2 to 9.8 per 1000 patient days. In 1995 only, hospital associated infections caused 88,000 demises, roughly one death every six minutes at a cost of $4.5 billion. Recently, in 2015, eighteen (18) babies mostly premature died within three months in Jamaica Hospitals from a nosocomial outbreak of *Serratia and Klebsiella spp.* on the neonatal ward out of forty-two (42) cases. There had been four nosocomial outbreaks since July 2015 of nosocomial bacterial infections acquired at the University Hospital of the West Indies and Cornwall regional Hospital in St. James [33].

The following associated variables have been credited to increase nosocomial rates: duration of hospital stay, indwelling catheter, mechanical ventilation,

mis-use of antibiotics, use of histamine (H₂) antagonists due to relative microbial

overgrowth, age and environmental conditions on ward. These issues, including

mis-escalation in the existence and severity of nosocomial infections. Nosocomial

urinary tract infections (UTI's), nosocomial surgical site infections (SSI's),

nosocomial pneumonia and nosocomial bloodstream infections (BSI's) all

account for 80% of hospital associated infections [50]. This statistics has not

changed considerably in the past 25 years. Infections by several pathogens have

developed into a primary nosocomial concern in the last decade, with a

considerable recent increase in associated illness and death [50].

The advent of multidrug-resistant (MDR) organisms have complicated the

challenge of treating these patients [19]. Limited studies have been done on this

topic in Trinidad and Tobago. Assessment has revealed that published studies

have been conducted only in one regional hospital over a decade ago. Of the four

publications retrieved, the scopes of the research studies were limited. These

studies were conducted on a: specific ward, particular type of hospital acquired

infection and particular type of nosocomial pathogen. There is therefore

paramount need to have more recent and frequently documented information on

nosocomial infections from a larger cross section of health care hospitals in

Trinidad and Tobago.

1.2 <u>Definition</u>

Nosocomial infection by definition refers to an infection occurring in a patient admitted on ward in a healthcare facility in which the infection was not present or incubating at the time of the patient's admission [15]. These infections are mainly the commonest problems encountered in patients admitted to healthcare facility, with approximately ten percent (10%) of warded patients developing some form of hospital associated infection. These infections occur 48 or more hours after the individual is admitted on ward without previous symptoms of the infection.

The absence of any predisposing factors or having a defensive factor does not essentially protect patients from acquiring nosocomial infections. There are numerous conditions that become more common with age. Some conditions become very common in elderly patients. The elderly patients are also often considered at risk due to reduce immune systems. Patients with reduced immune systems are at risk for developing nosocomial infection. Immune deficiency can arise as a medical condition, such as human immunodeficiency virus (HIV), diabetes mellitus or other chronic illnesses. Certain medications can also reduce immune functions including immune-suppressants, transplant patients and chemotherapy treatment for cancer [88].

4

There are many types of hospital acquired infections including: nosocomial respiratory tract infections, nosocomial urinary tract infections, nosocomial bloodstream infections, nosocomial skin and soft tissue infections and nosocomial central nervous system infections. As medical practices become more highly developed, the uses of intravascular catheters have become a criteria in the discipline of medicine and particularly frequent in the intensive care facilities (ICUs) where patients are seriously ill. These catheters provide a way to give high alert medications that are required to be given via a large vein and also serve as an instrument to assess the central venous pressure. Nosocomial blood stream infections resulting from central venous accesses are a rare type of nosocomial infections although; this type of hospital acquired infection is mainly avoidable when compared to the other types of hospital acquired infections. As with any other types of hospital acquired infections; nosocomial central venous catheter infections are related with increased expenditures in health care facilities.

Health care associated infections have been more potent and resistance more frequent to the antibiotics with MRSA being the most fatal type antibiotic-resistant bacteria. *Staphylococcus* associated health care infections have shown an increase in resistance to antibiotics from 22% in 1997 to more than 60% in 2007. The Centers for Disease Control and Prevention (CDC) approximates that

MRSA kills in the region of 19,000 patients annually. Prevalence of other multidrug-resistant bacteria are also rising, example vancomycin-resistant *Enterococci* (VRE) which, in 1997, was observed in about 15% of warded patients, a slight increase from about 1% in 1990. *Clostridium difficile* (*C. diff*), another important hospital acquired pathogen or bacteria, is also on the increase. The CDC estimates, there are 500,000 cases yearly in the United States, an increase from 150,000 cases in 2001 [48].

1.3 <u>Study Objectives</u>

The main objectives of this research were to conduct and provide accurate and authentic findings related to the epidemiological study of nosocomial infections at three regional tertiary hospitals in Trinidad. Specifically, the research study was designed at determining from the three regional tertiary hospitals the following objectives:

- Frequency of Nosocomial Infections (NIs) especially the urinary tract infections in Trinidad and Tobago.

- The frequency of multiple drug resistance among bacterial organisms associated with nosocomial infections in Trinidad and Tobago.

- Infection control measures practiced at the research hospitals.

- Cost of such nosocomial infections in terms of the morbidity and mortality.

1.4 **Justification of Study**

The information obtained from the above objectives will serve to give health care providers in the country the data that is needed to formulate policies and strategies that would be efficacious and effective in dealing with nosocomial infections and infection control measures.

Although limited studies have been carried out in Trinidad and Tobago on nosocomial infections, this present study will provide valuable information to stakeholders in both the public and private health sectors with respect to improvement in desired patient outcomes towards optimum health.

7

CHAPTER 2

2.0 Literature Review

2.1 Epidemiology

It has been discovered that hospital acquired infections (HAIs) are recurrent problems, identified chiefly in intensive care facilities. There are numerous findings by different researchers that have provided authentic information, be it in statistical or percentage ratings of nosocomial infections worldwide. These are as follows; in Europe, incidences vary from 1% for all types of nosocomial infections and up to 23.6% in pediatric ICUs (PICU) [28, 64]. Pediatric intensive care unit studies account for incidences between 6.1 - 15.1% [78] while others [66] in a cross sectional study reported a prevalence of 11.9% [25]. In the United States of America (USA), the Centers for Disease Control and Prevention (CDC) calculated approximately 1.7 million nosocomial infections from all types of microorganisms resulting in 99,000 deaths annually [32]. Other estimates designate two (2) million patients annually become infected with the yearly cost varying from $4.5 billion to $11 billion. In the United States of America (USA), nosocomial urinary tract infection (36%) is the most frequent type of nosocomial infection, followed by nosocomial surgical site infection (20%), then both nosocomial bloodstream and respiratory tract infection especially pneumonia (11%) infections [57]. In France, estimates of hospital acquired infection varied from 6.7% in 1990 to 7.4% [59]. At a national level, prevalence among patients

admitted on wards was 6.7% in 1996, 5.9% in 2001 and 5.0% in 2006. In 2006,

urinary tract infections (30.3%) were the most frequent type of nosocomial

infection followed by, pneumopathy (14.7%), nosocomial infections of surgery

site (14.2%), nosocomial infections of the skin and mucous membrane (10.2%),

other nosocomial respiratory infections (6.8%) and blood poisoning (6.4%) [7].

The nosocomial rates among adult patients in intensive care facilities were 13.5%

in 2004, 14.6% in 2005, 14.1% in 2006 and 14.4% in 2007 [62].

In Jamaica, eighteen (18) newborns died from forty two (42) cases from the

outbreak of infections that had occurred on the Neonatal Intensive Care Units at

the University of the Hospital of the West Indies and Cornwall Regional Hospitals

from June 2015 onwards. The outbreaks were caused by *Serratia* and *Klebsiella*

organisms through human contact, unsanitary environment and equipment [20].

Patients who acquire nosocomial infections are estimated to stay in the hospital

four (4) to five (5) additional days. During 2004-2005, an estimate number of

9,000 patients died annually with a hospital acquired infection, of which roughly

4,200 would have survived if, did not develop hospital acquired infections [79]. In

Italy, from 2000, estimates retrieve approximately 6.7% nosocomial infection rate

which resulted in 4,500 to 7,000 deaths [30]. A study conducted in Lombardy

produced a nosocomial infection rate of 4.9% of patients in 2000 [37]. In United

Kingdom, estimates showed a 10% nosocomial rate [5] with 8.2% approximated

in 2006. Switzerland predicts range varying from 2% and 14%. Rates were

expected at 8.5% of patients in 2005 in Finland [38]. In Belgium the prevalence of

hospital acquired infections is approximately 6.2%. Each year, about 125,500

patients are affected by a hospital acquired infection, causing approximately 3000

deaths. The additional expenses for the health insurance are predicted to be

roughly €400 million annually [21].

In Trinidad and Tobago information on nosocomial infections are lacking. Within

the period 1992-1995, Orrett, [52] documented that 7,158 hospital acquired

infections were observed from 72,532 patients. High nosocomial rates were

observed in the intensive care unit (ICU) (67/100), urology (30/100),

neurosurgery (29.5/100) and newborn nursery (28.4/100) wards. Nosocomial

urinary tract infections (4.1/100) accounted for the majority of nosocomial

infections (42%), followed by post-operative nosocomial wound infections

(26.8%) having a nosocomial rate of 2.6/100. That report by [52] estimated the

cost to the government of Trinidad and Tobago for nosocomial infections at a

whopping amount of 697,000 USD each year. The report further mentioned lack

of infection control management, poor hand-washing facilities, limited supplies,

absence of garbage cans on most wards and improvement of facilities were some

risk factors that contributed to a rise in the rate of hospital-acquired infections and

cross infections in the hospital environment [52]. Orrett indicated in [51] that, one

thousand three hundred and sixty (1,360) pediatric nosocomial tract infections

were identified from a total of twenty-six six hundred and three (26, 603)

admissions during a five (5) year retrospective chart review in a rural hospital.

The ages range from three (3) days to thirteen (13) years, with

10

46% boys and 54% girls. *Escherichia coli, Proteus mirabilis, Klebsiella spp.* and Group B *Streptococci* account for a total of 70% of all pathogens. The antibiotics with least effectiveness in increasing order for urinary tract infections were: Cephalexin, Ampicillin, Trimethoprim, Co-trimoxazole and Tetracycline whereas the most effective antibiotics were Nalidixic acid, Gentamicin and Amoxicillin-Clavulanic acid [51]. Orrett again reported that infection control actions designed at declining hospital acquired infections at the hospital are frequently disturbed by lack of concern of hospital administrators who seemingly are not aware of the high nosocomial infection rate [53]. The author stressed that strict observance to appropriate infection control practices and upgrading of health care facilities are vital steps in preventing cross infections in the health facilities.

Again in Trinidad and Tobago, from survey findings by [53], it indicated that one hundred and thirty nine (139) hospitals acquired infections were identified from six hundred and twenty nine (629) admissions to ICU. The nosocomial rate was 22.1% when compared to the general nosocomial infection rate of 15.3% for the whole health care facility. In the ICU, the main nosocomial infections were from the respiratory tract, 41 (29.5%), followed by surgical wounds, 35 (25.2%), urinary tract, 28 (20.1%) then bloodstream, 24 (17.3%). From 165 bacterial organisms, 80% of these organisms were gram negative bacilli, with *Pseudomonas aeruginosa*, 48 (36.6%), being the most common isolate followed

by *Klebsiella pneumoniae*, 27 (20.6%) then *Enterobacter sp*, 22 (16.8%). The major gram-positive isolates were *Staphylococcus aureus*, 23 (41.8%), *coagulase-negative Staphylococci*, 17 (30.9%) and *Enterococci*, 11 (20.0%). Of the twenty three (23) *Staphylococcus aureus* isolates, 15 (65.2%) were methicillin resistant *Staphylococcus aureus (MRSA)*. Eight (8) of the MRSA were from surgical wounds, five (5) from the respiratory tract specimens and two (2) from infected urine. Resistance to Ampicillin and Augmentin was soaring, 81.9% and 55.4%, correspondingly. Gentamicin, Aztreonam, Piperacillin-Tazobactam resistance rates were less than 15% [53]. These reports were from limited sources. There is therefore a need to have comprehensive documented information on nosocomial infection from a wider cross section of health care facilities in Trinidad and Tobago.

To be considered as a nosocomial infection, some factors will be associated and these includes: the patient ought to have been admitted for supplementary purposes than the hospital acquired infection and the patients too should have shown no indications of active or incubating infection. The location of a hospital acquired infection relies on the type of hospital procedures patients were given. Indications of hospital associated infections differ by the type of hospital associated infections of which include the following signs: inflammation, discharge, fever, and abscesses. Patients may experience pain and irritation at the infection site and many experience noticeable symptoms that can relate to any of the five ordinary types of nosocomial infections namely: nosocomial blood stream

infections, nosocomial urinary tract infections, nosocomial skin and soft tissue infection, nosocomial respiratory tract infection and nosocomial central nervous infection. These infections may lead to critical injury if patient lack proper medical care. In relation to each of the five ordinary types of nosocomial infections namely; Blood Stream Infections, Skin and Soft Tissue Infections, Urinary Tract Infections, Respiratory Tract Infections and Central Nervous System Infections, each will be discussed.

2.2 Nosocomial Bloodstream Infections

Nosocomial bloodstream infection (BSI) is a principal, infectious hurdle among seriously ill patients [42]. It represents about 15% of all hospital acquired infections [67, 81] and affects about 1% of all hospitalized patients [56] with an incidence rate of five (5) per 1,000 central line days [50]. The impact on patient outcome is critical and relates to the organization. Nosocomial BSI increases the mortality rate [73], extends patient stay in intensive care facilities (ICU) [13] and produces significant additional expenditures [65]. For these surveillances, prevention of nosocomial BSIs are high precedence and several infection control plans have been demonstrated to be successful [8, 9, 18 40, 43, 60, 70]. The Centers for Disease Control and Prevention (CDC) observation made descriptions of nosocomial BSI outline as two discrete entities: infections that are microbiologically documented, and those that are not, called clinical sepsis [23]. Although observation of the former can be laboratory based, surveillance of

clinical sepsis requires prospective on site observation. The observation approach establishes whether clinical sepsis will be noted thus affecting the entire nosocomial BSI incidence rate. Symptoms of nosocomial blood stream infections include: known organism in the blood and pathogen not associated with an infection at another site or with clinical features such as fever, chills and hypotension. Also, for microbiological documented BSI's, a communal skin contaminant is isolated from at least two blood cultures drawn on separate occasions from a patient with an intravascular device and if the doctor prescribed suitable antimicrobial treatment and a positive antigen test on blood [23].

Clinical sepsis was detected when the patient had fever, hypotension, or oliguria also called hypouresis (low output of urine) and inclusive of the following: blood not cultured, no micro-organism isolated and no apparent infection at another site and the doctor prescribed proper antimicrobial treatment for sepsis [23].

14

2.3 Nosocomial Skin and Soft Tissue Infection

This particular type of nosocomial infection, skin and soft tissue, include the clinical presentation of: pain, edema, warmth, erythema, violaceous bullae, cutaneous blood loss, skin sloughing, skin anesthesia, rapid evolution and gas in the tissue [11, 63]. Skin and Soft Tissue Infections (SSTIs), results from invasion of the skin and mostly occur due to trauma or surgery. Skin and soft tissue infections can be classified as simple, necrotizing or suppurative, [63]. Risk factors of acquiring skin and soft tissue infections include the following: older age, diabetes mellitus, immune-compromise, alcohol abuse and prolong hospitalization [82]. The prevalence of skin and soft tissue infections among in patient is estimated at 7% to 10% [83]. It is one of the most frequent infections among in patients with increased frequency among men [82]. Patients within the age range of 18 to 44 and blacks are more susceptible of acquiring skin and soft tissue infections. The following organisms: *Staphylococus aureus, Pseudomonas aeruginosa, Enterococcus* and *Escherichia coli* are commonly isolated from in patients associated with skin and soft tissue infections [44].

Management of skin and soft tissue infections is difficult owing to its variation of their presentation. The choice of antibiotic treatment may be inconsistent and inefficient. Site of care is dependent on the severity of skin and soft tissue infection: oral therapy is given to mild lesions whereas intravenous therapy is

administered to moderate to severe lesions. The duration of treatment is determined by constant monitoring and clinical judgement [82].

Penicillin is given as first line treatment for Group A *Streptococcus (Streptococcus pyogenes)* organisms identified from skin and soft tissue infections. Alternative treatments for *Streptococcus pyogenes* include: first generation Cephalosporin, Clindamycin, Macrolides, Glycopeptides or expanded spectrum Fluoroquinolones. For skin and soft tissue infections caused by Group B *Streptococcus (Streptococcus agalactiae)* organisms first line high doses of Penicillin G intravenously with Clindamycin are administered. Cephalosporins, beta-lactamase inhibitors, Carbapenem, Fluoroquinolones or Aminoglycosidesare given to treat the following organisms: *Klebsiella pneumoniae, Escherichia coli* and *Serratia marcescens* identified from in patients associated with skin and soft tissue infections [83]. First line anti-pseudomonal beta lactam combined with aminoglycoside treatments are given for *Pseudomonas aeruginosa* identified isolates associated with skin and soft tissue infections.

Patients with *Pseudomonas spp.* have mortality rates varying from 20% to 70% [1, 87].

16

2.4 Nosocomial Urinary Tract Infection (UTI)

Nosocomial UTI is produced by pathogenic infiltration of the urinary tract, resulting in an inflammatory response of the urothelium. Infections may be acute or chronic. The clinical indications of nosocomial urinary infections include: fever, chills, dysuria, urinary urgency, frequency and cloudy or redolent urine [34]. Gram negative bacteria are most often observed in hospital acquired urinary tract infections than Gram positive bacteria. *Escherichia coli* accounts for 75% to 95% of cases. Other gram-negative organisms namely; *Klebsiella, Proteus mirabilis, Enterobacter, Pseudomonas aeruginosa* and *Serratia* account for 40% of nosocomial urinary tract infections. Regarding gram-positive bacteria, *Staphylococcus saprophyticus* is observed in 5% to 10% of bacterial nosocomial urinary tract infections. Least frequent gram positive organisms associated with urinary tract infections are: *Enterococcus faecalis* and *Streptococcus agalactiae* [27].

Approximately 95% urinary tract infections occur when bacteria ascend the urethra to the bladder or ascend the ureter to the kidney. Nosocomial urinary tract infections accounts for being the most common that accounts for 40% of all types of hospital acquired infections. Nosocomial urinary tract infections have a rating of 15-20%. It is the most frequent cause of death among hospital associated infections and is the major cause of mortality in the intensive care facilities [27].

17

The main prevention of urinary tract infections is complete emptying of the bladder during urination. Increasing fluid intake, wiping front to back after defecation or antibiotic prophylaxis such as cephalexin 125 to 250 mg orally (po) once a day, Fosfomycin 3 g po for 10 days and Nitrofurantoin 50 or 100 mg once a day [27]. Treatments of urinary tract infections include antibiotics, surgery and to correct underlying structural abnormalities. The choice of antibiotic is dependent upon the patient's adherence history. First line treatment of infection of the bladder (cystitis) is Nitrofurantoin 100mg po twice daily for five (5) days and Trimethoprim/Sulfamethoxazole 10/800mg po twice daily for three (3) days or Fosfomycin 3g po once. Fluoroquinolones or β-lactam antibiotic are the given last resort. Phenazopyridine may help to control symptoms of dysuria until antibiotics do within the first 48 hours. Patients with inflammation of the urethra (urethritis) are given ceftriaxone 250mg IM with azithromycin 1g once daily or doxycycline 100mg twice daily for seven (7) days. For acute pyelonephritis (infection of the kidney and ureters) urinary infections; these patients are given ciprofloxacin 500 mg po twice daily for seven days and levofloxacin 750mg po once a day for five days. Another alternative is Trimethoprim/Sulfamethoxazole 160/800mg po twice daily for fourteen (14) days. First choice treatments are ciprofloxacin and levofloxacin. Other alternatives include; Ampicillin with Gentamicin, broad spectrum Cephalosporins example; Ceftriaxone, Cefotaxime, Cefepime, Aztreonam, Imipenem and Ampicillin/Sulbactam.

18

Piperacillin/Tazobactam are preferentially administered for patients with chronic pyelonephritis [27].

2.5 Nosocomial Respiratory Tract Infection

Nosocomial respiratory tract infections are major causes of extreme morbidity and mortality in United States of America hospitals, affecting probable five to ten of every 1,000 patients. Bacterial pneumonia accounts for 25% of all ICU infections. Ventilated acquired pneumonia is the highest in the initial course of hospital stay. Intubation and mechanical ventilation increases the risk of nosocomial respiratory infections [49]. Patients with critical underlying diseases are more susceptible of developing these infections and that risk is increased by exposure to respiratory therapy. According to Dixon, contaminated respiratory care devices were a major cause of infection [14]. Aspiration of nose and throat secretions is thought to be the most important cause of nosocomial respiratory infections. Dental plaque also might be a reservoir for bacteria in nosocomial respiratory infections [2]. Respiratory infections can be classified as bacterial pneumonia example ventilator- associated pneumonia and viral pneumonia example respiratory syncytial virus. Bacterial pneumonia infections are commonly due to gram negative bacilli (52%) and *Staphylococcus aureus* (19%) mostly of the MRSA type. *Haemophilus* spp. (5%) also is seen in respiratory infections. Respiratory infections are very frequent on the ICU ward and *Staphylococcus aureus* (17.4%), *Pseudomonas aeruginosa* (17.4%),

19

Klebsiella pneumoniae (18.1%), *Enterobacter* (18.1%)and *Haemophilus influenzae* (4.9%)are also commonly associated with nosocomial respiratory infections [46].

Concerning nosocomial respiratory tract infection, hospital acquired pneumonia is the second main type hospital associated infection. It prolongs a hospital admission by one to two weeks. Factors influencing nosocomial respiratory infections include; a) insertion site: subclavian or jugular sites, b) type: central tunneled, peripheral, c) material: teflon, silicon, polyurethane, PVC, polyethylene surface impregnated with silver, d) antibiotics, e) number of lumen: single-luminar, multiple- luminar and f) usage: drugs, nutrition, blood. Local signs of inflammation at the site of entry include; redness, tenderness, swelling, slight purulent exudate that is; prominent in peripheral lines and less in central lines. According to Liu, other systemic signs include; fever, rigors with no other source of fever greater than 37.8°C, clinical improvement after catheter removal, elevated inflammatory markers and typical pathogens in blood culture, purulent sputum, leukocytosis greater than 10.000 cells/µl [36].

Nosocomial respiratory infections can be treated with Erythromycin or Fluroquinolone for cases of legionellosis. The following antibiotics are also given when treating nosocomial respiratory infections: Amoxicillin with Clavulanic acid, Ceftazidime, Imipenem, Piperacillin/Tazobactam [49].

20

2.6 Nosocomial Central Nervous System Infection

Similar to the other types of nosocomial infections, infections involving the central nervous system are very serious too, if not life threatening. These infections can rise from superficial wounds, foreign bodies (ventricular shunts) and the deep structures of the brain parenchyma. The majority of nosocomial central nervous system is from bacterial meningitis and central nervous system shunt infections [45]. Forty per cent (40%) of bacterial meningitis infections are nosocomial [16]. The overall incidence is 0.56 per 10,000 hospital discharges. However, the rates are higher on pediatric services (3.3 per 10,000 discharges), high risk nurseries (2.1 per 10,000 discharges) and neurosurgical services (1.7 per 10,000 discharges). Within the years 1971 to 1974, National Nosocomial Infections Study (NNIS) reported rates of nosocomial central nervous system infections of ten (10) central nervous system infections per 100, 000 discharges. Additionally data in the years 1975 to 1982 revealed that the rate of nosocomial central nervous system was 84 per 100, 000 discharges [16].

Nosocomial central nervous system infections can be divided into surgical or device related and non-surgical related infections. The surgical or device-related infections are surgical site infections and can be further categorized into three groups: a) organ space infections, such as meningitis or ventriculitis; b) superficial infections involving the skin; or c) deep infections involving the brain.

21

Meningitis or ventriculitis is associated with ventriculostomies whereas superficial and deep skin and soft tissue infection with subarachnoid bolts, brain abscess, subdural empyemas, epidural abscess and meningoencephalitis with corneal or dural implants. Nosocomial meningitis can be associated with parameningeal infections and brain abscesses that occur after head trauma, neuroinvasive procedures, sepsis, high-risk neonates and immune-suppression [31]. Risks of acquiring nosocomial meningitis are due to neurosurgery and the presence of neurosurgical device. In most of recent studies published, from case reviews of nosocomial meningitis, gram negative (38%) was the more frequent organisms observed such as; *Escherichia coli* and *Klebsiella spp. Pseudomonas, Acinetobacter, Enterobacter* and *Serratia* organisms were least observed. Other organisms observed to cause nosocomial meningitis included: *Staphylococcus aureus,* coagulase negative *Staphylococci, Streptococcus pneumonia* and other *Streptococci* [39]. *Corynebacterium, Propionobacterium, Haemophilus, Listeria, Bacillus, Clostridium, Neisseria, Yersinia, Mycobacterium tuberculosis, Mycobacteria, Cryptococcus* and *Ascaris* organisms have too caused nosocomial shunt infections [45]. Vancomycin with Ceftazidime are both given to treat against gram negative bacilli such as *Pseudomonas spp.* and also gram positive organism *Staphylococcus aureus* [69].Tobramycin and Amikacin are given intrathecally to achieve effective therapeutic levels in the cerebrospinal fluid

22

(CSF) preferentially when treating against *Staphylococcus aureus* organisms.

Meropenem when administered parenterally, is also given to treat against

Pseudomonas organisms. Aztreonam has been proven to be very effective against

most gram negative organisms. Other alternative include the administration of

parenteral ciprofloxacin. Vancomycin is also given as an alternative for

Cloxacillin to treat against *Staphylococcus aureus* organisms [45].

2.7 Prevention and Control

Nosocomial Infections pose serious health problems or challenges to patient well-

being. Therefore, CDC provides world-wide guidance in close watch, outbreak

surveys, laboratory research and prevention of nosocomial infections. CDC uses

awareness acquired through these campaigns to spot infections and develop and

implement new plans to prevent and reduce nosocomial infections. Public health

action by CDC and other healthcare partners demonstrated great improvements in

clinical practice, medical methods and the continuing growth of infection control

guidance and prevention accomplishments.

It is advised that indwelling catheters be changed frequently, to prevent

persistence and reoccurrence of infection. At times, removal of catheter may

cause natural resolution of bacteriuria or asymptomatic cystitis.

With regards to ventilator which may be an aid to prevent the risk of hospital

acquired pneumonia infections, controlling hospital internal air quality needs to

be a fulfilled requirement at the most suitable areas. To an extent nosocomial

infections can be lessened to strengthen this point, an author cited Maryland's implementation which reported that; the State of Maryland employed the Maryland Hospital-Acquired Conditions Program which provided monetary rewards and consequences for individual hospitals based on their aptitude to prevent nosocomial infections. For first two years of the program, the nosocomial rates declined by 15.26%. The 15.26% reduction resulted in the health care system in Maryland saving more than $100 million with nosocomial UTI's, septicemia and pneumonia having the most savings. Should consistent outcomes be realized worldwide, the Medicare program would save approximately $1.3 billion during two years period and the health care system in entirety would save $5.3 billion [6].

Hospitals should comply with all sanitization protocols comprising uniforms, fumigating equipments, washing and other pre-emptive procedures. Proper hand washing along with usage of **alcohol rubs** by all health care staff prior to and after each patient contact is one of the most effective ways of fighting hospital associated infections. Cautious use of antibiotics is crucial. In spite of sanitation guidelines, patients can become susceptible of acquiring hospital associated infections. Patients are often given alternative antibiotics in controlling illness; that may amplify the **range** for the appearance of resistant strains. **In addition, sterilization is further than sanitizing; it destroys all pathogens on medical devices and surfaces via contact with chemicals, ionizing radiation, dry heat or steam**

under pressure. Safety measures are implemented to avoid spread of pathogens by regular paths in health care facilities.

Practicing of hand washing is the solitary way of minimizing the hazards of spreading skin pathogens between patients or from one spot to another on the same patient. Frequent hand washing as often between contacts with patients and after contact with blood, body fluids, secretions, excretions, and equipment or items infected by these agents is a vital constituent of infection management and isolation preventative measures. The transmission of hospital associated infections, among immune-compromised patients is linked with health care staff's hand infectivity in nearly 40% of cases, and is a difficult predicament in the modern health care facilities. The most appropriate application for staffs to conquer this challenge is performing proper hand-hygiene actions. This is why the World Health Organization (WHO) initiated in 2005, the Global Patient Safety Challenge [85]. The objective of hand sanitation is to eradicate the transitory flora with proper act of hand washing, with various types of soap; customary and antibacterial and alcohol-based gels. The major challenges observed in the performance of hand sanitation are associated with the inadequacy of sinks, lengthy time and act of hand washing procedures. A simple way in resolving this issue can be using alcohol-based hand rubs, since, it is a quicker process in contrast to accurate hand washing [26].

25

Gloves too have a significant function in minimizing the risks of spread of pathogens. In essence gloves are worn for these important purposes in health care facilities. They give a protective barrier to avoid gross infectivity of the hands when contacting blood, body fluids, secretions, excretions, mucous membranes and non-intact skin. In the United States, the Occupational Safety and Health Administration have authorized wearing gloves to lower the risk of blood borne pathogen associated infections [22].

As with other preventative and control methods, the wearing of gowns can also be regarded to offer effective protection. It restricts infectious substances off clothing. In contrast to other studies, two (2) recent researches validate that staff gowning in the neonatal intensive care facility is a needless practice [54, 74].

Wearing gowns did not minimize neonatal colonization, infection or mortality rates. There was no change in traffic patterns on the ward or in hand washing behavior [54] and it was not cost effective [72].The widespread use of gloves and gowns was observed to be no superior than the use of gloves alone in averting rectal colonization by Vancomycin-resistant *Enterococci* in a medical intensive care facility .

Furthermore, some health personnel have challenged the idea that the stethoscope, may essentially be a path for transmission of nosocomial infections.

26

In a research of a hundred and fifty (150) health care staffs, fifty (50) paramedics, fifty (50) nurses, and fifty (50) doctors, *Staphylococcus* species; mostly coagulase negative were cultured from 89% of the participant's stethoscopes with the average amount of colony forming units increased, when the stethoscopes were not sanitized [29]. In general, 48% of health care workers cleaned their stethoscopes each day or week, 37% each month, 7% annually and 7% had never cleaned them. Cleaning the stethoscope caused an immediate decline in the bacterial count by 94% with alcohol swabs, 90% with a non-ionic detergent, and 75% with antibacterial soap [29].

There are no researches on the valuable outcome of frequently cleaning stethoscopes on hospital associated infection rates. Nonetheless, it is advised that habitual disinfection should be done at least once per day, as the intensity of infectivity increases from 0% to 69% following each additional day without cleaning of the stethoscope [68]. Isopropyl alcohol is an effective cleaning agent [41] but may desiccate the stethoscope's rubber seals and spoil the tubing if used regularly.

Human pathogens, *S. marcescens* are involved also in hospital acquired infections (HAI's) particularly catheter-associated bacteremia, urinary tract, wound and respiratory infections for 14% of HAI. *Serratia* is commonly found in the RTI & UTI of hospitalized adults and in the gastrointestinal system of children.

27

Outbreaks of infection initiated by *S. marcescens* have been reported quite frequently. Study of epidemiologic markers is important in an endeavor to trace the cause of infection or to avoid patient-to-patient transmission. Numerous techniques have been outlined for the typing of *S. marcescens* including serotyping, phage typing, biotyping, bacteriocin typing, whole cell protein fingerprinting and plasmid analysis[55,71]. Of the techniques, majority were not adequately sensitive to discriminate different subtypes. In the preceding years, there has been substantial interest publicized in using rRNA as a probe to detect polymorphisms in bacterial chromosomal DNA. This technique, ribotyping, has been used for epidemiologic studies of many bacterial species, including *Serratia marcescens*. It was found to be more discriminating when compared to biotyping, serotyping, and bacteriocin typing and has an equivalent discriminative power compared with total DNA analysis. However, the use of ribotyping in clinical microbiology laboratories has been limited because of the technical challenges and prolonged time needed for Southern blot analysis. Recently, a novel DNA fingerprinting strategy centered on the PCR amplification of variable length chromosomal series with a variation of primers was reported.

One of these methods, identified as random amplified polymorphic DNA assay, is established on the usage of simple random primers in a polymerase chain reaction of low stringency to enlarge sections of the genome and has been practiced efficaciously for the typing of numerous microbial species [86].

On the other hand [80] used consensus primers in the polymerase chain reaction to augment DNA series localized between sequential repetitive elements, such as the 126-bp enterobacterial repetitive intergenic consensus (ERIC) sequence in gram negative bacteria and strongly suggested this method to be likely for subtyping gram negative enteric bacteria.

CHAPTER 3

3.0 Methodology

3.1 <u>Study Design</u>

This research was a Cross Sectional Study conducted at three major hospitals in Trinidad and Tobago namely; Eric Williams Medical Sciences Complex (EWMSC), San Fernando General Hospital (SFGH) and Port of Spain General Hospital (POSGH) over twelve (12) months study period from June 1st 2013 to May 31st 2014.

Ethics approvals were granted to conduct the research study at the three regional hospitals from the University Campus Ethics Committee and the three Regional Health Authority Ethics Committees.

According to World Health Organization (WHO), health care associated infection (HCAI) is defined as: "An infection occurring in a patient during the process of care in a health-care facility which was not present or incubating at the time of admission. This includes infections acquired in the hospital but appearing after discharge and also occupational infections among staff."

31

At each of the study sites, confirmed cases of all types of nosocomial infections were identified on the research wards at each of the research hospitals on separate days of the week via the World Health's Organization definition of nosocomial infection, clinical symptoms and laboratory diagnosis of nosocomial infections. Each week, prospective cases of nosocomial infections were reviewed from doctor's notes in patient's dockets.

Patients notes were written in their charts by the doctors attending to them for any clinical signs of nosocomial infections three days (72hrs) for all types of nosocomial infections following their date of admission on ward with the exception of nosocomial blood stream infections (BSI) of which was observed two days (48hrs) following patients date of admission.

The standard criterias that were used along with WHO's definition to confirm nosocomial cases were: the patient had no growth of organism from laboratory culture present at day one of their admission and no signs and symptoms present at day one of admission of temperature spikes, worsening coughing or dyspnea (shortness of breath) or tachypnea (rapid breathing), bronchial rates, breath sounds, vomiting, fever, leukopenia <4000, low white blood cell (WBC) counts or leukocytosis 1200 WBC/mm, sloppiness at wound, redness, swelling, warmth, hotness around wound area, septicemia, hypotension (low blood temperature), dysuria (painful urination), urgency and super tenderness.

32

A total of 2600 patient dockets for the duration of the research period were obtained at each of the research hospitals and reviewed for prospective cases of nosocomial infections. Each patient docket was examined weekly at each of the research hospital to ascertain the nosocomial infection status of each patient. The extrapolated data from the patient dockets were entered on separate data collection sheets for each nosocomial patients and was analyzed using SPSS version 20. Descriptive statistics was used to analyze graphs and frequency tables for data presentation and inferential statistics was used for estimation and hypothesis testing. Variables measured included: age, gender, causative pathogen and type of nosocomial infection. Codes were assigned for the nosocomial patient's names on the data collection sheets. In addition, the nosocomial patient's names, their laboratory numbers and the dates of when their samples were sent to the laboratories by doctor or nurse in charge were used to trace in the log book for their sample number which helped to distinguish the respective nosocomial isolates from the other isolates. The nosocomial isolates were confirmed by standard laboratory and biochemical tests. Samples were sent day one of patient's admission to confirm that the patients had no growth of organism present at day one of their admission. Following day three of patient's admission for all types of nosocomial infection with the exception of nosocomial blood stream infection which was two days following patient's admission; the researcher reviewed patient's notes written by responsible doctor for any clinical symptoms of nosocomial infection by WHO's definition and criteria.

3.2 <u>Target Population</u>

The study population was all patients hospitalized on the following wards: Medical, Surgical, Pediatrics, Intensive Care Unit (ICU) and Obstetrics & Gynecology in public hospitals in Trinidad during the period June 1st, 2013 to May 31st, 2014 for at least one day.

3.3 <u>Sample Size Calculation</u>

The sample size was calculated via a Cluster Sampling method by wards of patient's files, the most practical sampling approach and via the World Health Organization definition and standard criterias for NIs, prospective nosocomial cases were selected from the defined population.

Surveillance was conducted on a weekly basis for fifty two (52) weeks for prospective nosocomial cases and patient's nosocomial laboratory bacterial isolates were obtained during the research period from June 2013 to May 2014. The average confirmed number of nosocomial cases by WHO's definition recovered from each week's surveillance was two (2).

Therefore, via cluster sample size calculation: number of wards multiplied by number of surveillance days multiplied by average number of HAI patients confirmed during each week's surveillance.

That is; 5 wards x 52 surveillance days x 2 = 520 patients were expected to acquire nosocomial infection during the data collection period.

Hence, 520 patients from clustered sample size calculation were expected to have been associated with nosocomial infections with confidence interval of 95% and relative precision of 10% within the research period.

3.4 Inclusion and Exclusion Criterias

All patients with features suggestive of nosocomial infections who were willing to participate and who gave their written or verbal consent on ward were included in the study. All such in patients with features of nosocomial infections who refused to participate were excluded. All ethnic and gender groups of the population were included in the study. There were no biased approaches or selection of subjects in the study. Minors and pregnant women were included in the study because as in patients they form an integral part of in patients who were taken care of in the hospital. They were equally exposed to any risk factor for developing hospital acquired infection hence; any plans to prevent such risk factors should also involve them. Minors were included after obtaining oral or written informed consent from the parents or guardians or head nurse in charge of ward. Out-patients from Accident & Emergency Wards and Renal Wards were excluded from this research study as infections from these type patients were considered community acquired infections.

3.5 <u>Laboratory Diagnosis</u>

Bacterial isolates were collected by the responsible doctors on ward and sent to the laboratory at each of the research sites for identification. Standard tests including gram staining and biochemical tests were performed on the recovered isolates to identify them from urine, blood, tracheal, sputum, wound swab, stool and cerebrospinal fluid specimens. Manual Antimicrobial Susceptibility Testing too was performed using agar disk diffusion method for all bacterial isolates on Mueller Hinton agar as recommended by Clinical and Laboratory Standards Institute (CLSI) [47, 84]. For each drug, indication was made on the recording sheet whether the zone size is susceptible (S), intermediate (I) or resistant (R) based on the interpretation chart.

An alternative susceptibility test was the MicroScan Automated Antimicrobial Susceptibility Testing which was more specific in naming the organism unlike the Agar Disk Diffusion method which was manual, less costly and more timing consuming. The MicroScan system provides automated bacterial identification and susceptibility testing with traditional methods. The system processes conventional panels in seconds, simplifying identification and susceptibility testing while standardizing result. Susceptibility results were entered on each of the patient's questionnaire form then computed in Microsoft excel file then into SPPS files for analysis.

36

Assessment of the infection control measures practiced at the research hospitals and mortality figures were reviewed and assessed from patient's dockets. In addition, total admission figures for all in-patients admitted on all the research wards were retrieved each month from the medical record unit at each of the research hospitals which was used to calculate the nosocomial rate.

Polymerase Chain Reaction (PCR)

The ten (10) most frequently occurring nosocomial pathogens: *Serratia marcescens,* which were recovered from the nosocomial outbreak, were further analyzed. These isolates were identified by standard and biochemical tests. Their susceptibilities to the following antibiotics; Amikacin (AK), Aztreonam (ATM), Ceftazidime (CAZ), Cefepime (FEP), Ciprofloxacin (CIP), Gentamycin (GM), Piperacillin/Tazobactam (TZP), Tetracycline (TE), Tobramycin (TOB) and Tigecycline (TGC) were regulated by agar disk diffusion antimicrobial susceptibility method also known as Kirby-Bauer disk antibiotic testing according to the procedures suggested by the Clinical and Laboratory Standards Institute.

The use of this ERIC based PCR Finger-printing technique was applied in studying the clinical isolates of *Serratia* from hospitalized patients. This approach was compared with conventional system, such as antimicrobial susceptibility profile [61].

PCR-based typing molecular method was used to differentiate band patterns of clinical *Serratia marcescens* isolates cultured on separate blood agar plates and

incubated at 35·C for 24-48 hours and inoculated into Brain Heart Infusion (BHI)

tubes containing glycerol and stored in freezer at -70·C for PCR typing method.

The PCR-based typing method was done by the DNeasy Blood and Tissue

Handbook [58]. The extracted DNA (0.1, ug) or supernatant fluid (1ul) was added

to a reaction mixture overlaid with mineral oil. The reaction mixture and oil had

previously been exposed to shortwave UV light for ten (10) minutes to cross-link

any contaminating DNA to prevent its acting as a template for the reaction.

Primers used were ERIC1 (5'-GTGAATCCCCAGGAGCTTACAT-3') and

ERIC2 (5'-AAGTAAGTGACTGGGGTGAGCG3'). The reaction mixture (100-

,lA volumes) contained 1 U of Taq polymerase, 10 mMTris (pH 8.3), 50 mMKCl,

2.5mM $MgCl_2$, 0.01% (wt/vol) gelatin, 250 puM(each) deoxynucleoside

triphosphates and 1 puM single primer.

Amplification was performed in a PHC-3 thermal cycler, with temperature

ramping as follows: 95°C for five (5) minutes to denature template; four low,

stringency cycles of 94°C for one (1) minute, 26°C for one (1) minute,72°C for

two (2) minutes; 40 cycles of 94°C for 30 seconds, 40°C for 30 seconds, and

72°C for one (1) min and lastly, 72°C for ten (10) minutes.

Negative controls were prepared, with no addition of template DNA.

Amplification products (10pA) were isolated by agarose gel electrophoresis in

1.6% agarose gels in Tris-borate-EDTA buffer containing ethidium bromide

38

(1 pLg/ml), at 30 V for 6 hours, and visualized by UV trans-illumination [35, 61, 77].

In addition, all samples were prepared and examined on at least three separate occasions. The PCR patterns were considered to be matching on the basis of comparable numbers and matching locations of all major bands. Small alterations in the intensities of faint bands were disregarded. From the PCR typing technique and antimicrobial susceptibility profile testing, nosocomial patients were placed on treatment plans and were equally monitored to determine the outcome of their treatments including the infection control measures instituted during their management.

39

CHAPTER 4

4.0 Results

From a total of 126,668 admissions to the study sites; 450 cases of nosocomial

infections were identified during this one year prospective cross sectional study

within the period of June 2013 to May 2014. Research Site B accounted for

having sixty three (63) hospital acquired infections from a total of 39,950

admissions. In contrast, Research Site A was observed to have a total of two

hundred and sixty five (265) nosocomial infections from a total of 48,057

admissions while Research Site C had one hundred and twenty two (122) hospital

acquired infections from a total of 38,661 admissions during the research period.

4.1 <u>Incidence of Nosocomial Infections in Trinidad and Tobago 2013 – 2014</u>

The research period was from June 2013 to May 2014 (52 weeks). Surveillance

was conducted once weekly on separate days at the three (3) research sites. There

were fifty two (52) surveillance days and an average of fifty (50) dockets were

reviewed for prospective cases on the research wards on separate days at the three

(3) research sites. In calculating the incidence; the number of surveillance days

(52) was multiplied by the average number of dockets reviewed each surveillance

(50) day from all the research wards; Surgical, Medical, Pediatrics, Intensive Care

Unit (ICU) and Obstetrics & Gynecology. Therefore, 52 Surveillance days

multiplied by 50 (average files reviewed during each surveillance day) equal 2600

cases reviewed at each research site multiplied three (3) equal 7800 files reviewed in total at the three research sites during research period and four hundred and fifty (450) nosocomial cases were recovered during the research period from all three research sites. The incidence of all three (3) regional hospitals was calculated by dividing number of confirmed cases over total number of reviewed files multiplied by one hundred; (450/7800) x 100 = 5.8%. Therefore incidence was 5.8% for in-patients associated with nosocomial infections at all three regional hospitals.

Incidence at Site A

This incidence was calculated by dividing the number of hospital associated cases (265) recovered within the research period by the total files reviewed (2600) multiplied by 100 which equaled to 10.2%.

Incidence at Site B

Similarly, Research Site B's incidence was calculated by dividing the number of hospital associated cases (63) recovered during the research period by the total files reviewed (2600) multiplied by 100 which equaled to 2.4%.

Incidence at Site C

Research Site C's incidence was calculated by dividing the number of hospital associated cases (122) recovered within the research period by the total files reviewed (2600) multiplied by 100 which equaled to 4.7%.

41

4.2 <u>Nosocomial Rates in Trinidad and Tobago 2013 – 2014</u>

The nosocomial rate was calculated by dividing the number of nosocomial cases recovered during the research period by the total number of patients admitted on the research wards multiplied by a 100. The number of patients admitted on research wards for all three regional hospitals was 126,668 and the total number of nosocomial cases recovered for the research period was 450. Hence nosocomial rate for research period was; 450/126,668 x 100 = 0.36%; 3.6 per 1000 patients.

The nosocomial rate for Research Site A was 265/48057 = 0.55%; 5.5 per 1000 whereas the nosocomial rate for Research Site C was 122/38,661= 0.32%; 3.2 per 1000 patients, half less than that of Research Site A's nosocomial rate. In contrast the nosocomial rate for Research Site B was the least of all observed at the three (3) regional hospitals; 63/39950 = 0.16%; 1.6 per 1000 patients, which was one third of the nosocomial rate when compared to Research Site A's nosocomial rate.

Table 1 shows the frequency distribution of nosocomial infections among the three research sites during the study period. A total of 450 nosocomial cases were observed during the research period of which Research Site A accounted for having the most number of hospital acquired associated cases (265) being the largest of the three research regional hospitals followed by Research Site C having (122) number of nosocomial cases. Research Site B (63) had the least amount of nosocomial infections during the research period.

Table 1:- Frequency Distribution of Nosocomial Infections in Trinidad and Tobago 2013 – 2014

Research Site Hospitals	Frequency of NI's	Total Admission at
Site A	265	48057
Site B	63	39950
Site C	122	38661
Total	450	126668

Table 2 reflects the frequency distribution of gender cases. Male patients (251) were predominantly more associated with nosocomial infections than female patients (199). Fifty six (56%) of nosocomial infections were observed from the male gender which was significant indicating that males were more susceptible to developing hospital acquired infections than female patients of which accounted for (44%) being associated with nosocomial infections. The difference between male and female figures was not statistically significant.

Table 2:- Frequency Distribution of Demographic Variables

Gender	Number of Nosocomial Cases (n)	%	P- Value
Male	251	56	1.960
Female	199	44	1.960
Total	450	100	

44

Table 3: Calculation of T- Test

	Male	Female
Number of observations	251	199
Mean = Sum of Gender (X) values / N(Number of values)	125.60	99.49
Standard Deviation $$S=\sqrt{\frac{\sum(X-M)^2}{n-1}}$$ © easycalculation.com	72.79	57.65
Variance = s^2	5298.04	3324.49

To calculate t,

1) subtract the mean of the second group from the mean of the first group

99.49 – 125.60 = 26.11

2) calculate, for each group, the variance divided by the number of observations minus 1

45

Male :

$[5298.04/ (251-1)] = [5298.04 /(250)] = 21.19$

Female:

$[3324.49/ (199-1)] = [3324.49/ (198)] = 16.79$

3) add the results obtained for each group in step two together

21.19+16.79=37.98

4) take the square root of the results of step three

square root of 37.98=6.16

5) divide the results of step one by the results of step four

26.11/6.16=4.24

To interpret the results,

f) calculate the degrees of freedom

g) look up the value in the table

h) interpret the value of t

46

Degrees of freedom

The degree of freedom for the t-test is calculated by adding up the number of observations for each group, and then subtracting the number one (because there is one group). For example, $(199 + 251 - 1) = 449$

Distribution of T

The values of t are printed in tables in most statistics texts. The values of the degrees of freedom are listed in a column down the side, and the values of alpha are listed in a row across the top. There are different tables for one-tailed and two-tailed tests of t.

Find the correct table for the number of tails. Then find the intersection of the degrees of freedom and the value of alpha (p-value) in the table. That value is the value that the calculated t-score must equal or exceed to indicate statistical significance.

For a one-tailed test of t, with df=449 and p=.05, t must equal or exceed 1.645.

For a two-tailed test of t, with df=449 and p=.05, t must equal or exceed 1.960.

47

Table 4: Two Tailed test table

degrees of freedom	significance level					
	20%	10%	5%	2%	1%	0·1%
1	3·078	6·314	12·706	31·821	63·657	636·619
2	1·886	2·920	4·303	6·965	9·925	31·598
3	1·638	2·353	3·182	4·541	5·841	12·941
4	1·533	2·132	2·776	3·747	4·604	8·610
5	1·476	2·015	2·571	3·365	4·032	6·859
6	1·440	1·943	2·447	3·143	3·707	5·959
7	1·415	1·895	2·365	2·998	3·499	5·405
8	1·397	1·860	2·306	2·896	3·355	5·041
9	1·383	1·833	2·262	2·821	3·250	4·781
10	1·372	1·812	2·228	2·764	3·169	4·587
11	1·363	1·796	2·201	2·718	3·106	4·437
12	1·356	1·782	2·179	2·681	3·055	4·318
13	1·350	1·771	2·160	2·650	3·012	4·221
14	1·345	1·761	2·145	2·624	2·977	4·140
15	1·341	1·753	2·131	2·602	2·947	4·073
16	1·337	1·746	2·120	2·583	2·921	4·015
17	1·333	1·740	2·110	2·567	2·898	3·965
18	1·330	1·734	2·101	2·552	2·878	3·922
19	1·328	1·729	2·093	2·539	2·861	3·883
20	1·325	1·725	2·086	2·528	2·845	3·850
21	1·323	1·721	2·080	2·518	2·831	3·819
22	1·321	1·717	2·074	2·508	2·819	3·792
23	1·319	1·714	2·069	2·500	2·807	3·767
24	1·318	1·711	2·064	2·492	2·797	3·745
25	1·316	1·708	2·060	2·485	2·787	3·725
26	1·315	1·706	2·056	2·479	2·779	3·707
27	1·314	1·703	2·052	2·473	2·771	3·690
28	1·313	1·701	2·048	2·467	2·763	3·674
29	1·311	1·699	2·043	2·462	2·756	3·659
30	1·310	1·697	2·042	2·457	2·750	3·646
40	1·303	1·684	2·021	2·423	2·704	3·551
60	1·296	1·671	2·000	2·390	2·660	3·460
120	1·289	1·658	1·980	2·158	2·617	3·373
$\propto$	1·282	1·645	1·960	2·326	2·576	3·291

48

Interpret the value of t

If the calculated t-score equals or exceeds the value of t indicated in the table, then the researcher concluded that there is a statistically significant probability that the relationship between the two variables exists and is not due to chance. In this example, the computed t-score of 4.24 is smaller than the table value of t, so there is no relationship between female and male. Hence, the difference is not statistically significant between male and female.

49

Table 5 features the total admission per hospital facility for each of the research sites during the research period from June 2013 to May 2014. Intensive Care Unit (272) had the lowest number of admissions for all three research sites. Medical facilities at Research Site A (15573) had the largest number of admissions followed by Research Site B (11042) and Research Site C (8570) having the least number of admissions for the Medical Facilities. On the contrary, Research Site C (18329) had the most number of admissions for Pediatrics followed by Research Site A (9004) then Research Site B (5425). Research Site A had the largest number of admissions for Surgical (11212) and Obstetrics & Gynecology (12268) facilities followed by Research Site B having the second largest amount of admission for Surgical (11684) and Obstetrics & Gynecology (11795) facilities. Research Site C had the least number of admissions on the Surgical (5807) and Obstetrics and Gynecology wards (5687). The total admissions for each research site were used to calculate the nosocomial rate. The number of admissions on the medical, pediatrics and surgical facilities were significant as these wards tend to have the most cases of nosocomial infections due to more in-patients and longer hospital stay.

50

Table 5:-Total Admissions on Research Wards at the Research Sites during Study Period

Research Wards	Research Sites				
	A	**B**	**C**	**Total**	**%**
Surgical	11212	11684	5807	28703	22.6
Medical	15573	11042	8570	35185	27.8
Pediatrics	9004	5425	18329	32758	25.9
ICU	0	4	268	272	0.2
Obst. & Gyn.	12268	11795	5687	29750	23.5
Total Adm	48057	39950	38661	126668	100

Table 6 depicts frequency distribution of nosocomial infections within age groups. Age group 60 and above category accounted for having the highest frequency of nosocomial infections of a hundred and twenty (120) which was significant amongst the other age groups. Nosocomial patients within the age 0-9 had the second largest frequency of infection (108) followed by patients within the age 50-59 having a total of (64) then age group 40-49 having a total of fifty-three (53) infections. Age group 30-39 was observed to have a total of forty-nine (49) infections followed by age group 20-29 having a total of forty (40) infections. Patients within the age group 10-19 had the least number of nosocomial infections with a total of sixteen (16) nosocomial infections during the twelve months (12) research period.

Table 6:- Age Distribution of the Patients with Nosocomial Infections

Age Group	Total NI'S (n)	%
0-9	108	24
10-19	16	3.6
20-29	40	8.8
30-39	49	10.9
40-49	53	11.8
50-59	64	14.2
60 and above	120	26.7
Total	450	100

Table 7 is showing frequency distribution of nosocomial infections at research sites. Surgical wards (152) had the most numbers of nosocomial infections 33.8 % followed by Medical facilities (120) then Pediatrics (94) health facilities followed by Intensive Care Unit (ICU) (82). Obstetrics & Gynecology (2) ward had the least amount of nosocomial infections (0.4%) during the research period. From findings, number of nosocomial infections on surgical wards (152) was significant. Patient skin preparation in the operating room, usage of chlorhexidine- based preparations, fore-arm antisepsis, hair removal, surgical attire are vital factors to consider for safe procedures when carried out on the surgical wards so as to reduce the nosocomial rate on the surgical ward.

Table 7:- Frequency Distribution of nosocomial infections on research wards in Trinidad and Tobago 2013 – 2014

Wards Hospitals	Frequency of NIs (n)	Total Admissions at
Surgical	152	28703
Medical	120	35185
Pediatrics	94	32758
ICU	82	272
Obstetrics & Gynecology	2	29750
Total	450	126668

54

Table 8 shows the frequency distribution of the types of nosocomial infections with Skin and Soft Tissue Infections (SSTI) (168) being the most frequent type of nosocomial infections 37.3% then Blood Stream Infections (128) followed by Urinary Tract Infections (90) then Respiratory Tract Infections (58). Central Nervous System Infections (6) was the least frequent type of nosocomial infections observed, 1.3%.

Table 8:- Distribution of Types of Nosocomial Infections in Trinidad and Tobago 2013-2014

Type of Infection	Value	%
Skin & Soft Tissue	168	37.3
Blood Stream	128	28.4
Urinary Tract	90	20.0
Respiratory Tract	58	13.0
Central Nervous System	6	1.3
Total	450	100

55

Table 9 shows the distribution of nosocomial infection in each month of the research period. The month of August (54) had the highest number of nosocomial infections which was significant followed by March having (48) nosocomial infections then November accounted for (45) nosocomial cases. The month of June (21) had the least number of nosocomial infections.

Table 9:- Distribution of Nosocomial Infections in Trinidad and Tobago by Month, 2013 - 2014

Month	Frequency of NI's	Total Adm. at Research Sites	%
June	21	10345	4.7
July	22	11242	4.9
August	54	10861	12
September	40	11011	8.9
October	40	10574	8.9
November	45	10195	10
December	29	9718	6.4
January	42	10929	9.3
February	44	10372	9.8
March	48	10056	10.7
April	30	10605	6.7
May	35	10760	7.7
Total	450	126668	100

56

Table 10 shows the frequency of microorganisms that were associated with nosocomial infections during the study period. *Staphylococcus spp (193)* followed by *Pseudomonas aeruginosa* (109) accounted for the most frequent causative organism that was associated with nosocomial infections. These organisms were the most common multi drug resistant organisms producing many strains. *Acinetobacter spp* (101) and *Klebsiella spp* (100) nosocomial frequencies were very significant too. On the contrary, unlike *Staphylococcus spp (193)* and *Pseudomonas aeruginosa* spp. (109), the following nosocomial pathogens were not as commonly associated with nosocomial infections within the study period: *Providencia stuartii (14)*, *Stenotrophomonas maltophilia* (14), *Streptococcus spp (10)*, *Citrobacter koseri* (6), *Alcaligenes spp.* (6), *Morganella morgannii* (4), *Burkholderia (P) cepacia* (4) and *Achromobacter xylosidans* (1) of which was the least frequent, 0.1%. Multiple organisms were mostly identified in each of the nosocomial cases accounting for eight hundred and fifty nine (859) nosocomial pathogens associated in all the nosocomial cases.

57

Table 10:- Distribution of Identified Organisms associated with HAI in Trinidad and Tobago 2013 -2014

Identified Organisms	Frequency	%
Staphylococcus spp	193	22.4
Pseudomonas aeruginosa	109	12.7
Acinetobacter spp	101	11.8
Klebsiella spp	100	11.6
Enterobacter spp	74	8.6
Enterococcus spp	64	7.4
Escherichia coli	58	6.8
Candida albicans	58	6.8
Proteus sp	22	2.6
Serratia spp	21	2.4
Providencia stuartii	14	1.6
Stenotrophomonas maltophilia	14	1.6
Streptococcus spp	10	1.2
Citrobacter koseri	6	0.7
Alcaligenes spp	6	0.7
Morganella morgannii	4	0.5
Burkholderia (P) cepacia	4	0.5
Achromobacter xylosoxidans	1	0.1
Total	859	100

58

Table 11 shows the susceptibility patterns of the nosocomial organisms.

Staphylococcus spp. had the most susceptibility patterns (15) which were very significant indicating that more than one strains of the same organism existed.

Table 11: - Susceptibility Pattern of *Staphylococcus spp.* in Trinidad and Tobago 2013- 2014

Staphylococcus spp. (193/859)

Antibiotics

	RD	TGC	VA	CXM	E	Ox	Tob	SXT	CN	LZP	CIP	Fox	AMC	AML	CEC	GM	CAZ	TE
a)	S	S	S	R	R	R	R	R	R	R	R	R	R	R	R	R	R	R
b)	S	S	S	R	R	R	R	R	S	R	R	R	R	R	R	R	R	R
c)	S	R	S	R	R	R	R	R	R	R	R	R	R	R	R	R	R	R
d)	S	S	S	R	R	R	R	R	R	S	R	R	R	R	R	R	R	R
e)	S	R	S	S	S	R	R	R	R	R	R	R	R	R	R	R	R	R
f)	S	R	S	S	R	R	R	S	R	R	S	R	R	R	R	R	R	R
g)	S	R	S	R	S	R	R	S	R	R	S	R	R	R	R	R	R	R
h)	R	R	R	R	S	S	S	S	R	R	R	R	R	R	R	R	R	R
i)	S	R	S	S	S	R	R	S	R	R	S	S	S	R	R	R	R	R
j)	S	S	S	R	R	R	R	R	R	R	R	R	R	R	R	R	R	R
k)	S	S	R	R	R	R	R	R	R	R	R	R	S	R	R	R	R	R
l)	S	S	S	R	R	R	R	R	R	R	R	R	R	R	R	R	R	R
m)	R	R	S	R	S	S	R	S	R	R	S	R	S	R	S	S	R	R
n)	R	R	R	R	S	R	R	R	S	R	S	S	R	S	S	S	S	S
o)	S	R	S	R	S	R	R	S	R	R	S	S	S	R	R	S	R	S

59

Table 12 represents the susceptibility pattern of *Pseudomonas aeroginosa* organism which had four different patterns indicating that four different strains of the same organism existed.

Table 12: - Susceptibility Pattern of *Pseudomonas aeroginosa* in Trinidad and Tobago 2013- 2014

Pseudomonas aeroginosa (109/859)

Antibiotics

	IPM	TZP	CAZ	CIP	CN	GM	ATM	ETP	ATM	TOB
a)	S	S	S	S	S	R	R	R	R	R
b)	S	S	S	S	R	S	R	R	S	R
c)	S	S	S	S	S	R	R	S	R	R
d)	R	S	S	S	R	S	S	R	R	S

Table 13 represents the antibiogram profile of *Acinetobacter spp.* indicating that five distinct strains of the same organism existed. The following antibiotics were observed to be most frequently resistant to *Acinetobacter spp.*: AML, AMC, ATM, CEC, ETP, CXM, GM and TE.

Table 13: - Susceptibility Pattern of *Acinetobacter* in Trinidad and Tobago 2013- 2014

Acinetobacter (101/859)

Antibiotics

	CAZ	CIP	ETP	SXT	TZP	IMP	TG	TOB	AK	COL	TGC	FEP	CN	AML	AMC	ATM	CEC	ETP	CXM	GM	TE
a)	S	S	S	S	S	S	R	R	R	R	R	R	R	R	R	R	R	R	R	R	R
b)	S	R	R	S	R	S	S	R	R	R	R	R	R	R	R	R	R	R	R	R	R
c)	R	R	R	R	R	S	R	S	S	S	S	R	R	R	R	R	R	R	R	R	R
d)	R	S	R	S	S	S	R	R	R	R	R	S	S	R	R	R	R	R	R	R	R
e)	S	S	S	S	S	R	R	R	R	R	R	R	R	R	R	R	R	R	R	R	R

61

Table 14 shows the susceptibility of *Klebsiella spp.* indicating that six (6) different strains of the same organism existed.

Table 14: - Susceptibility Pattern of *Klebsiella spp.* in Trinidad and Tobago 2013- 2014

Klebsiella spp. (100/859)

Antibiotics

	CN	IPM	TZP	AMC	FEP	CAZ	CXM	TOB	CIP	LEV	TE	ETP	F	NOR	GM	SXT	AML	CEC	GN	ATM	TGC
a)	S	S	S	S	S	S	S	S	S	S	R	R	R	R	R	R	R	R	R	R	R
b)	R	S	R	R	R	R	R	R	R	S	S	R	R	R	R	R	R	R	R	R	R
c)	R	S	S	R	R	R	R	R	S	R	R	S	S	S	R	R	R	R	R	R	R
d)	R	S	S	S	R	R	R	R	S	R	R	S	R	S	R	S	R	R	S	R	R
e)	S	S	S	R	R	R	R	S	R	R	R	R	R	R	R	R	R	R	R	R	R
f)	S	R	S	S	S	S	R	R	S	R	R	R	R	R	R	R	S	R	R	S	S

62

Table 15 represents the susceptibility of *Enterobacter spp.* indicating that five different strains of the same organism existed. CAZ, CIP, ETP AND SXT were mostly susceptible whereas the following antibiotics AK, FEP, CN and TE were most frequently resistant to *Enterobacter spp.*

Table 15: - Susceptibility Pattern of *Enterobacter* in Trinidad and Tobago 2013- 2014

Enterobacter (74/859)

Antibiotics

	CAZ	CIP	ETP	SXT	TZP	TOB	IMP	GM	ATM	CXM	AK	FEP	CN	TE
a)	S	S	S	S	S	R	S	R	R	R	R	R	R	R
b)	S	S	S	S	S	S	S	R	R	R	R	R	R	R
c)	S	S	S	S	S	R	S	S	S	S	R	R	R	R
d)	S	S	R	R	S	S	R	S	R	R	S	S	R	R
e)	S	S	R	R	S	R	R	R	S	R	R	S	S	S

63

Enterococcus spp. had three different susceptible patterns as displayed in table 16 inferring that three different strains of the same organism existed. CIP, CT, CN and AK were the most resistant antibiotics.

Table 16: - Susceptibility Pattern of *Enterococcus spp.* in Trinidad and Tobago 2013- 2014

Enterococcus spp. (64/859)

Antibiotic

	CEC	CXM	AMC	ETP	TZP	IPM	CAZ	CIP	CT	CN	AK
a)	S	S	S	R	R	R	R	R	R	R	R
b)	R	R	R	S	S	S	R	R	R	R	R
c)	R	S	R	R	R	S	S	S	S	S	S

64

Table 17 represents three susceptibility patterns of *Escherichia coli* inferring that three different strains of the same organism existed.

Table 17: - Susceptibility Pattern of *Escherichia coli* in Trinidad and Tobago 2013- 2014

Escherichia coli (58/859)

Antibiotics

	CK	CN	SXT	AMP	AMC	AML	ATM	CEC	CAZ	CIP	E	ETP	GM	IPM	TZP	FEP	TGC
a)	S	S	S	S	S	R	R	R	R	R	R	R	R	R	R	R	R
b)	R	R	S	R	S	S	S	S	S	S	S	S	S	S	S	R	R
c)	R	R	R	R	R	S	S	R	R	R	R	R	R	R	S	S	S

Table 18 represents no susceptibility pattern for *Candida albicans spp.* as these organisms were antifungals and tend to be non-susceptible to antibiotics due to their pharmacodynamics properties as they are fungus and are not susceptible to antibiotic treatments.

Table 18: - Susceptibility Pattern of *Candida albicans* in Trinidad and Tobago 2013- 2014

Candida albicans (58/859)

Non- Susceptible

65

Table 19 represented two susceptibility patterns for *Proteus spp.* indicating that two strains of the same organism existed.

Table 19: - Susceptibility Pattern of *Proteus spp.* in Trinidad and Tobago 2013- 2014

Antibiotic Profile of Proteus spp. (22/859)										
Antibiotic										
CAZ	CIP	CN	TZP	AMC	CEC	GM	IPM	NOR	F	SXT
a) S	S	S	S	R	R	R	R	R	R	R
b) R	R	R	S	S	S	S	S	S	R	R

Table 20 represents seven (7) susceptible patterns of *Serratia marsescens* organismsindicating that seven (7) different strains of the same organism existed.

Table 20: - Susceptibility Pattern of *Serratia spp.* in Trinidad and Tobago 2013- 2014

Serratia spp. (21/859)

Antibiotic

	ATM	CAZ	FEP	CIP	CN	TZP	TE	AK	TOB	AML	AMC	CEC	SXT	GM	TGC	CT	LEV	IMP	PIP	ETP
a)	S	S	S	S	S	S	S	R	R	R	R	R	R	R	R	R	R	R	R	R
b)	S	S	S	S	R	S	S	S	S	R	R	R	R	S	R	R	R	R	R	R
c)	S	S	R	S	R	S	R	R	R	R	R	R	S	S	R	R	R	R	R	R
d)	S	R	R	R	R	R	S	R	R	R	R	R	R	R	R	R	R	R	R	R
e)	S	S	S	S	R	S	S	R	R	R	R	R	S	S	R	R	R	R	R	R
f)	S	S	R	S	R	S	R	R	R	R	R	R	S	S	R	S	R	R	R	S
g)	R	R	S	R	R	R	R	R	S	R	R	R	S	R	R	R	S	S	S	R

Table 21 represents one susceptibility pattern for *Providencia stuartii spp.* indicating that one strain of the organism existed.

Table 21: - Susceptibility Pattern of *Providencia Stuartii* in Trinidad and Tobago 2013- 2014

Providencia stuartii (14/859)			
Antibiotic			
AK	TGC	MEM	
a) S	S	S	

68

Table 22 shows two (2) different susceptibility patterns of the *Stenotrophomonas maltophilia spp.* inferring that two (2) different strains of the same organism existed.

Table 22: - Susceptibility Pattern of *Stenotrophomonas maltophilia* in Trinidad and Tobago 2013- 2014

Stenotrophomonas maltophilia (14/859)

    Antibiotic

    AK TGC MEM CAZ LEV SXT

	AK	TGC	MEM	CAZ	LEV	SXT
a)	S	S	S	R	R	R
b)	R	R	R	S	S	S

69

Table 23 represents one (1) susceptibility pattern for *Streptococcus spp.* inferring that one strain of the organism was present.

Table 23: - Susceptibility Pattern of *Streptococcus spp.* in Trinidad and Tobago 2013- 2014

Streptococcus (10/859)

Antibiotic

   GM TZP MEM CAZ FEP

	GM	TZP	MEM	CAZ	FEP
a)	S	S	S	S	S

Table 24 shows two (2) susceptibility patterns of the *Citrobacter koseri* organism indicating that two (2) strains of the organism existed.

Table 24: - Susceptibility Pattern of *Citrobacter koseri* in Trinidad and Tobago 2013- 2014

Citrobacter koseri (6/859)

Antibiotic

   SXT TZP F NOR AMC CEC CXM CN CIP ATM CAZ GM TOB AMP TE

	SXT	TZP	F	NOR	AMC	CEC	CXM	CN	CIP	ATM	CAZ	GM	TOB	AMP	TE
a)	S	S	S	S	S	S	S	S	S	R	R	R	R	R	R
b)	R	S	R	R	R	R	R	R	S	S	S	S	S	R	R

70

Table 25 represents two (2) susceptibility patterns of the *Alcaligenes spp.* indicating that two strains of the organism existed. CAZ, CIP and TZP were the most frequently susceptible antibiotics for *Alcaligenes spp.*

Table 25: - Susceptibility Pattern of *Alcaligenes* in Trinidad and Tobago 2013- 2014

Alcaligenes spp. (6/859)

Antibiotics

   CAZ CIP TZP SXT TOB CN TE

	CAZ	CIP	TZP	SXT	TOB	CN	TE
a)	S	S	S	S	R	R	R
b)	S	S	S	R	S	S	S

Table 26 represents one (1) susceptible pattern inferring that only one (1) strain of the *Morganella morgannii* organism was present.

Table 26: - Susceptibility Pattern of *Morganella morgannii* in Trinidad and Tobago 2013- 2014

Morganella morgannii (4/859)

Antibiotic

   ATM FEP CIP GM IPM TZP

	ATM	FEP	CIP	GM	IPM	TZP
a)	S	S	S	S	S	S

71

Table 27 shows one (1) susceptible pattern inferring that *Burkholderia (P)* *cepacia* had only one strain of the organism present.

Table 27: - Susceptibility Pattern of *Burkholderia (P) cepacia* in Trinidad and Tobago 2013- 2014

Burkholderia (P) cepacia (4/859)

Antibiotic

	CAZ	FEP	TZP	TGC	TOB	SXT	AK	CIP	GM	TE
a)	S	S	S	S	S	S	R	R	R	R

Table 28 shows *Achromobacter xylosoxidans* having no susceptible pattern.

Table 28: - Susceptibility Pattern of *Achromobacter xylosoxidans* in Trinidad and Tobago 2013- 2014

Achromobacter xylosoxidans (1/859)

Non- Susceptible

72

Table 29 shows the distribution of nosocomial pathogens obtained as outbreak isolates during the research period. *Serratia* species (10) occurred as an outbreak during the study from the NICU and among nosocomial Blood Stream Infections. This occurred over a two month period (October 1 – November 30, 2013) and warranted further analysis. Other isolates that were obtained included: *Klebsiella spp.* (5), *Escherichia coli* (1), *Acinetobacter* (2), *Pseudomonas spp.* (3), *Staphylococcus spp.* (16) of which eight (8) were methicillin resistant coagulase negative *Staphylococcus* species. *Enterococcus* (1), *Enterobacter spp.* (6) and *Alpha hemolytic Streptococcus* (1) were also identified via standard and biochemical tests during the nosocomial outbreak.

The *Serratia* isolates were used via DNeasy Blood and Tissue Handbook (Qiagen, 2006) in the ERIC based PCR Finger-printing typing molecular technique to identify the band patterns. Five distinct band patterns were identified and five different susceptibility patterns were identified too from the same clinical *Serratia marcescens* isolates inferring that five (5) different strains of the same organism were present during the outbreak.

73

Table 29:- Antibiogram Characteristics of Outbreak- Related Isolates of *Serratia marcescens* in Trinidad and Tobago 2013 - 2014

{Serratia spp. frequency - (10/45)}

Ward	Age	AK	ATM	CAZ	FEP	CIP	GM	TZP	TE	TOB	CN	AML	AMC	CEC	TG	Band Patterns	Outcome
1) NICU	28wks	R	S	S	S	S	R	S	S	R	S	R	R	R	S	III	Still warded
2) NICU	44wks	S	S	S	S	S	S	S	S	S	R	R	R	R	R	I	Discharged
3) NICU	35wks	S	S	S	S	S	S	S	S	S	R	R	R	R	R	I	Discharged
4) NICU	28wks	S	S	S	S	S	S	S	S	S	R	R	R	R	R	I	Discharged
5) NICU	41wks	S	S	R	R	R	R	R	R	R	R	R	R	R	R	IV	Still warded
6) NICU	3wks	R	S	S	S	S	R	S	S	R	S	R	R	R	R	II	Discharged
7) NICU	8days	R	S	S	S	S	R	S	S	R	S	R	R	R	R	II	Discharged
8) NICU	35wks	R	S	S	R	S	S	S	S	R	R	R	R	R	S	V	Died
9) NICU	8days	R	S	S	R	S	S	S	S	R	R	R	R	R	S	V	Still warded Cub 1
10) NICU	28wks	R	S	S	S	S	R	S	S	R	S	R	R	R	S	III	Still warded Cub III

74

PCR Findings

Figure 1 below displays the results obtained from polymerase chain reaction

(PCR) base typing molecular method. The amplification products were separated

via 1.6% agarose gel electrophoresis molecular method and viewed under ultra

violet trans-illumination. Five (5) different band patterns were observed from all

the clinical *Serratia marsescens* isolates and one band pattern was contaminated.

The two ends are 1 kilo base ladder and within the ladders are the ten *Serratia*

marsecens strains encoded 1-10 following that respective order which were

recovered from the outbreak. The occurrence of this outbreak of *Serratia*

marsecens was unknown.

75

Ladder   1   2   3   4   5   6   7   8   9 10 Ladder

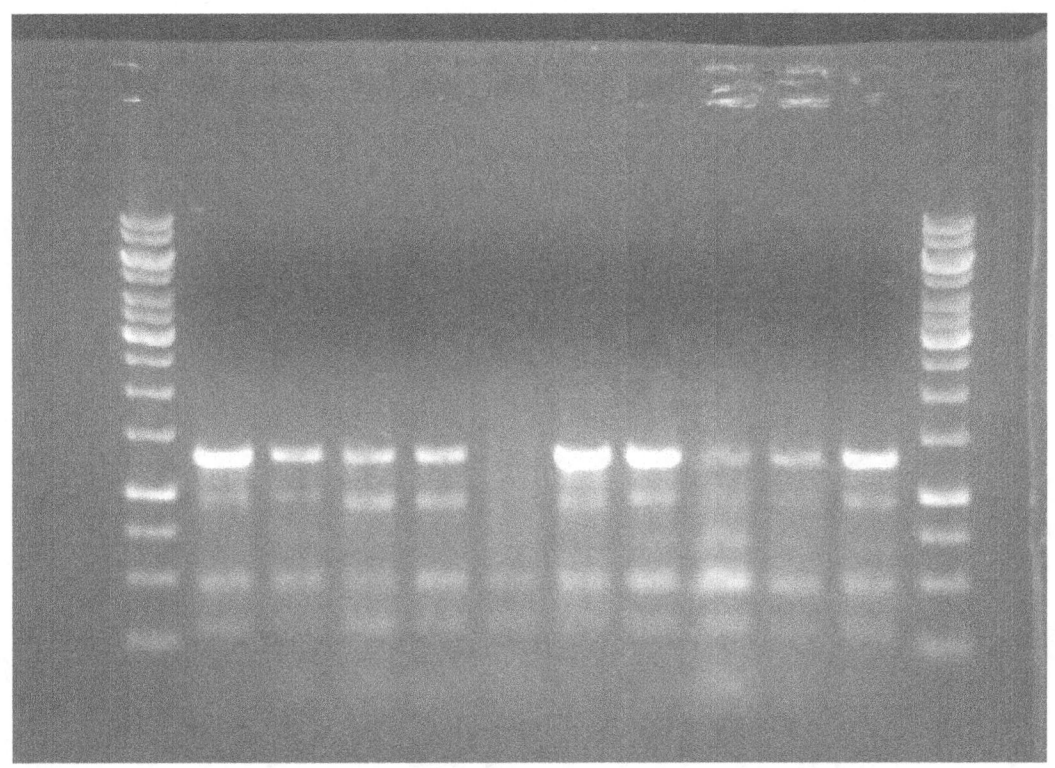

Figure 1:- Photo Showing PCR Band Patterns of *Serratia marsescens* Isolates

From Figure 1 above:

1) The two ends represent the 1 kilo base ladders.

2) The lanes numbered one (1) – ten (10) represent the *Serratia marcescens* organisms in chronological order.

3) Lanes 2, 3 and 4 represents band pattern 1.

4) Lanes 6 and 7 represents band pattern 2.

5) Lane 5 represents pattern 4.

6) Lanes 1 and 10 represent band pattern 3.

7) Lanes 8 and 9 represent band pattern 5.

Significant Findings

a). The incidence was 5.8% for all research sites. The incidence at Site A was the highest (10.2%) followed by Site C having a nosocomial incidence of 4.7%. Site B had the least nosocomial incidence of 2.4%.

b). The nosocomial rate was 3.6 per 1000 patients for all three hospitals and 5.5 per 1000 patients at Site A, 3.2 per 1000 patients at Site C and 1.6 per 1000 patients at Site B.

c). Four hundred and fifty (450) nosocomial cases were accounted for from a total of 126,668 admissions at all three (3) research sites. .

d. Site A (265) had the largest frequency of nosocomial infections followed by Site C (122) then Site B (63).

e. Neonatals (108) and patients 60 and above (120) had the highest nosocomial frequencies.

f. Surgical (152) and Medical (120) wards had the greatest number of nosocomial infections whereas Obstetrics and Gynecology (2) facility had the least frequency of nosocomial infection.

g. Skin and soft tissue infections (168) and blood stream infections (128) were the most prevalent types of nosocomial infections observed. On the contrary,

nosocomial Central nervous system infections (6) were observed to be the least frequent.

h. *Staphylococcus spp.* (193) and *Pseudomonas aeroginosa spp. (109)* had the highest nosocomial frequencies whereas *Citrobacter koseri (6), Alcaligenes (6), Morganella morgannii (4), Burkholderia (P) cepacia (4) and Achromobacter xylosidans (1)* were the least observed nosocomial pathogens.

i). Fifteen different susceptibility patterns were accounted for *Staphylococcus spp.* indicating that fifteen (15) different strains of the same nosocomial pathogen existed.

j). Clinical *Serratia marcescens* were mostly observed from the outbreak on the NICU facility of which accounted for having five (5) different susceptibility patterns and five (5) different PCR band patterns indicating that five (5) different strains of the same organism existed from the ten (10) recovered isolates.

k). The *S. marcescens* nosocomial pathogens were observed to be mostly resistance to Amoxicillin (AML), Amoxicillin/Clavulanic acid (AMC) and Cefaclor (CEC). The following antibiotics however: Aztreonam (ATM), Ceftazidime (CAZ), Cefepime (FEP), Ciprofloxacin (CIP), Piperacillin/Tazobactam (TZP), Tetracycline (TE) and Amikacin (AK) were observed to be very frequently susceptible to *S. marcescens* isolates.

l). The occurrence of the *S. marcescens* outbreak was unknown which resulted in sixteen nosocomial infections; twelve (12) BSIs, (50% being females and 50% males), two (2) nosocomial SSTIs from two female adult patients 71 and 42 of years respectively on surgical 7 ward, one (1) Nosocomial Respiratory Tract Infection from pediatric surgical ward and one (1) Nosocomial Urinary Tract Infection from a 65 year old male patient on the surgical 6 septic ward.

m) Of the *S. marcescens* nosocomial pathogens; fifteen (15) were identified as *Serratia marcescens* with the exception of one (1) isolate which was identified as *Serratia fonticola* via standard and biochemical tests.

n) From the outbreak; five (5) of the patients were treated and discharged and four (4) remained hospitalized on wards under treatment and one (1) death was reported from the outbreak that had occurred between the months of October 2013 and November 2013.

o) Of the 450 nosocomial cases retrieved from patient dockets during weekly surveillance at the three (3) regional research sites; three (3) patients were transferred to another ward, one (1) patient was discharged against medical advice, fourteen (14) patients were discharged and re-admitted or transferred to an alternative health care facility, eighty three (83) patients were reported to be still warded (hospitalized) under treatment (medical care) and sixty patients (60) were noted to have been discharged.

p) From the total nosocomial cases (450) observed during the research period at the three regional research sites, thirty (30) deaths resulted from these cases.

81

CHAPTER 5

5.0 Discussion

5.1 Research Findings

The calculated incidence of nosocomial infection from research findings was 5.8% for all the three (3) regional hospitals. The incidences at each of the three (3) regional hospitals were as follows: Research Site A; 10.2%, Research Site B; 2.4% and Research Site C; 4.7% respectively of which was similar to other developing countries. The incidence at Research Site A (10.2%) was lesser when compared to Benin; another developing country whose incidence was 19.1%, [76]. There were other developing countries that had similar variations and some incidences were higher than the Research Site's incidences for example, the incidence varied between 2.5% and 14.8% in Algeria, Burkina Faso [12] Senegal [24] and the United Republic of Tanzania [3]which was two times greater than the average European's incidence; 7.1% reported by the European Centre for Disease Prevention and Control [17].The actual burden of nosocomial infections is expected to be even more in hospitals with frailer substructures and rarer resources. Additionally, the rates in developing countries were much higher than in developed countries, where they range from 5-10%, [4, 7].

82

According to Coignard [7], he established that there is an urgent need to implement feasible and sustainable approaches towards hospital acquired infection through the means of prevention, surveillance and control in developing countries. In accordance to the ratings of the three regional research sites, the findings of each are as follows: at Site A, this research site had the most nosocomial infections; two hundred and sixty five (265) during the research period followed by Site C having one hundred and twenty two (122) cases of hospital associated infections then Site B had the least number of nosocomial infections; sixty three (63) during the research period.

The age of patients who had NIs ranged from eight (8) days old to ninety- six (96) years old with males being more predominant (56%) when compared to the female gender (44%). The frequency of nosocomial cases garnered from neonates was the second highest (108) inferring that these patients were more susceptible of acquiring nosocomial infections owing to their weak immune system. Neonatals were more susceptible of acquiring nosocomial infections owing their weak immune system therefore they may acquire colonization of any organism. Babies require more handling hence the spread by contact. Frequency of nosocomial cases amongst elderly in patients 60 and over years old, were the highest (120) due to risk factors of changes in their non-adaptive immunity, chronic diseases, medications, malnutrition, and functional impairments. Strausbaugh, [75] indicated that the T-lymphocyte production and proliferation declined with age which results in decreased cell-mediated immunity and

decreased antibody production to new antigens. Neonatals accounted for 24% of all nosocomial infections whereas patients sixty and over were observed to have 26.7% frequency of all nosocomial cases.

Of the hospital facility, surgical wards had the highest nosocomial infections (152) followed by Medical wards (120) then Pediatrics wards (94) then Intensive Care Unit (82). Obstetrics & Gynecology (2) had the least number of nosocomial infections. Despite the considerable effort devoted to observe each ward, it is of vital importance that key focus be placed on the surgical, medical and pediatric facilities where the nosocomial cases were highest. Another aspect of great interest is; special attention should be invested in sterilizing surgical tools, frequent hand washing and changing of gloves as often as possible.

The month of August (54/10861) was observed to have the highest number of nosocomial infections followed by March (48/10056). The month of June (21/10345) however, was observed to have the least number of nosocomial infections.

The researcher made further discoveries of nosocomial Skin and Soft Tissue Infections (168/450) being the most frequent type of nosocomial infections observed then nosocomial Blood Stream Infections (128/450) followed by nosocomial Urinary Tract Infections (90/450) then nosocomial Respiratory Tract Infections (58/450). Nosocomial infections from the Central Nervous System (6/450) were the least frequent type of nosocomial infection observed within the

research period. The amount of Skin and Soft Tissue nosocomial infections were significant. David, [10] reports that Skin and soft tissue infections account for 15% of all nosocomial infections chiefly among surgical patients being the most frequent type of nosocomial infection. Similarly, the researcher observed Skin and soft tissue infections being the most frequently observed type nosocomial infection accounting for 37.3% of all nosocomial cases.

The frequent spread of hospital acquired infections is primarily by direct contact hence, Skin and Soft Tissue Infections being the most common type of nosocomial infections observed from research findings.

Staphylococcus spp. (193/859) and *Pseudomonas aeruginosa* (109/859) organisms were one of the principal gram positive and gram-negative nosocomial pathogens respectively connected with hospital acquired infections during the research period. The cumulative occurrence of multi-drug-resistant *Staphylococcus spp.* and *Pseudomonas aeruginosa* strains were alarming as effective antibiotic choices were severely limited. Other frequently associated multi drug resistant nosocomial organisms included *Acinetobacter spp.* (101/859) and *Klebsiella spp.* (100/859).

Klebsiella and *Staphylococcus spp.,* were the most frequently observed causative organisms in nosocomial blood stream infections and *Proteus spp., Alcaligenes spp.* and *Achromobacter xylosoxidans* where the least commonly observed causative organisms in nosocomial blood stream infections whereas *Candida*

albicans, *Enterobacter* and *Escherichia coli isolates* were most commonly observed in nosocomial urinary tract infections.

Identified Organisms

Of the 859 nosocomial organisms, 73.7% of isolates were gram negative rods with *P. aeruginosa*, 109 (12.7%), being the predominant gram negative nosocomial pathogen followed by *Acinetobacter*, 101 (11.8%) then *Klebsiella sp*, 100 (11.6%). The main gram positive isolates were *Staphylococcus spp.* *(193/859)* (22.5%) and *Enterococci spp.* 64/859 (7.5%) and *coagulase negative Staphylococci*, 50/859 (5.8%). Of the *Staphylococcus spp.* (193/859), 88/859 (10.2%) were methicillin resistant *Staphylococcus aureus* (MRSA) and 55/859 (6.4%) were methicillin resistant coagulase negative *Staphylococcus*.

Types of Nosocomial Infections

Nosocomial Skin and Soft Tissue Infections (SSTI) and Blood Stream Infections (BSI) were the most common types of nosocomial infections with occurrences of 37.3% and 28.4% respectively. Nosocomial infections were commonly transmitted via direct contact hence Skin and Soft Tissue Infections being the most frequent type of hospital acquired infection observed. Respiratory tract infections (RTI) and blood stream infections (BSI) were observed to be most frequently associated on the medical facilities. Also, BSIs were notably mostly observed on the pediatric medical facilities whereas Skin and Soft Tissue

86

Infections (SSTI) were most frequently observed on the surgical wards. Nosocomial central nervous system infections and nosocomial urinary tract infections were more commonly observed on the medical wards followed by surgical wards. Nosocomial urinary tract infections were least observed on the gynecology wards.

Susceptibility Patterns of Antibiotics

Of the susceptibility test results; Amoxicillin (AML), Amoxicillin/Clavulanic acid (AMC), Cefaclor (CEC), Cefuroxime (CXM), Ampicillin (AMP) and Trimethoprine/Sulphamethazole (SXT) were observed of being the most frequently resistant antibiotics. Resistance of these antibiotics were commonly observed for the following nosocomial pathogens: *Acinetobacter, Klebsiella, Staphylococcus, Enterobacter, Escherichia coli, Serratia spp.* and *Citrobacter koserii* organisms. However; the nosocomial pathogens were frequently susceptible to the following antibiotics: Imipenem (IMP), Piperacillin/Tazobactam (TZP), Ceftazidime (CAZ), Ciprofloxacin (CIP), Gentamicin (GM), Clindamycin (CN), Aztreonam (ATM), Levofloxacin (LEV), Linezolid (LZD), Piperacillin (PIP), Meropenem (MEM), Tetracycline (TE), Colistin sulphate (CT), Tigercycline (TGC), Nitrofurantoin (F), Ertapenem (ETP), Cefepime (FEP), Norfloxacin (NOR), Amikacin (AK) and Tobramycin (TOB). *Pseudomonas aeruginosa, Acinetobacter* and *Klebsiella* were observed to be most frequently susceptible to Imipenem, Amikacin, Ciprofloxacin, Gentamicin and

87

Cefepime. Quinupristin (QD) was observed to be most commonly susceptible for *methicillin resistant coagulase negative Staphylococcus (MRCNS)* organisms and Clindamycin, Rifamficin, Tigercycline, Vancomycin and Linezolid were also commonly observed to be effective for *methicillin resistant coagulase negative Staphylococcus (MRCNS)* isolate.

Sulphamethazole was frequently observed to be susceptible for *Citrobacter koserii*, *Stenotrophomonas maltophilia* and *Alcaligenes* sp. In contrast Sulphamethazole was least susceptible for *Burkholderia (P) cepacia* isolates. In-patients were more likely of being associated with nosocomial infections due to; inconsistency in sanitizing work areas, lack of proper ventilation on some wards, irregularity in changing long term use of invasive devices such as urinary and central venous catheters, long term stay in hospitals and previous hospitalization exposure. Patients acquired nosocomial infections either endogenously or from external environment (exogenously). Endogenous nosocomial infections were as a consequence of opportunistic pathogens residing in or on external surfaces of patients and brought on by conditions present at or as a direct outcome of events on the wards. In contrast, exogenous hospital acquired infections were the result of pathogens being transmitted by patients as they are shed from numerous thresholds of exit while the patients were hospitalized.

88

Nosocomial Blood Isolates

Forty-five (45) nosocomial blood isolates were recovered with *Serratia*

marcescens, being the most frequent (10). The following isolates were also

recovered: *Klebsiella spp.* (5), methicillin resistant coagulase negative

Staphylococcus spp. (8), *Escherichia coli* (1), *Acinetobacter* (2), *Pseudomonas*

spp. (3), *Staphylococcus* (7), *Epidermidis aerogenes* (2), *Enterococcus* (1),

Enterobacter spp (5) and *Alpha hemolytic Streptococcus* (1).

PCR of *Serratia marcescens* Isolates

ERIC Polymerase chain reaction (PCR) base-typing molecular method was used

to further analyze *Serratia marcescens* organisms from the outbreak. The ERIC1

and ERIC2 primers successfully typed all isolates examined via PCR -based

typing. Five distinct band patterns and five (5) distinct susceptibility patterns were

observed from all the clinical *S. marcescens* (10) isolates recovered. The

occurrence of this outbreak of *Serratia marcescens* was the result of the spread of

five strains of the same organism on the neonatal wards. No potential

environmental sources of infections was identified. However, *S. marcescens*

survives well in moist hospital environments. Nosocomial epidemics of *Serratia*

marcescens infections have been ascribed to contaminated disinfectants,

intravenous solutions, mechanical ventilators, nebulizers, arterial pressure

monitors, urine-measuring containers and other medical equipments. It was noted

that ERIC PCR – based finger-printing was particularly suitable for reviewing the

epidemiology of nosocomial *S. marcescens* pathogens. This rapid typing method facilitated the prompt and sensitive assessment of disease epidemic so that effective preventive measures can be instituted if common sources are identified.

Control Measures Practiced at Institutions

The infection control measures practiced at the health care facilities as recorded from patient's dockets during weekly surveillance included: isolation of MRSA patients. These type patients were separated from other patients so as to avoid non-affected patients of becoming contaminated and wearing of gloves and masks were also observed to be practiced by the barrier nurses when attending to MRSA patients. Other infection control measures that were observed and written in patient's dockets that were practiced at the health care facilities included: strict observance of contact precaution. Ventilatory support, antibiotics, analgesia, fluid resuscitation and frequent cleaning of infected wound with lysol were also observed from notes from patient's dockets during surveillance as some of the infection control practices done at the research sites.

90

CHAPTER 6

6.0 Conclusion and Limitation

6.1 <u>Conclusion</u>

The objectives of this research study were attainable.

- The incidence was 5.8% for all three regional hospitals. Site B had the lowest incidence (2.4%) inferring that good infection control management was practiced. On the contrary site A had the largest incidence (10.2%) whereas site's C's incidence was (4.7%).

- The nosocomial rate was 3.6 per 1000 patients for all three research sites. Individually, Site A's nosocomial rate was 5.5 per 1000, 3.2 per 1000 for Site C and 1.6 per 1000 for Site B. Site B the lowest nosocomial rate.

- Majority of the nosocomial infection were observed at Site A (265). Site B (63) has the least number of nosocomial infections whereas Site C accounted for one hundred and twenty two (122) nosocomial infections.

- Males (251) were more associated with nosocomial infections when compared to female (199) in-patients.

91

- Neonatals (108) and in patients sixty (60) years and above (120) accounted in having the highest nosocomial frequencies.

- Surgical (152) and Medical (120) facilities accounted for the highest number of hospital acquired infections inferring that activities performed on these wards be closely monitored to reduce the nosocomial frequencies.

- Skin and soft tissue (168) and blood stream (128) infections were the most frequent type of nosocomial infections whereas central nervous system infection (6) was the least frequent type of nosocomial infections observed.

- *Staphylococcus* spp. (193), *Pseudomonas*spp.(109), *Acinetobacter* spp. (101), *Klebsiella* spp. (100) were the most frequently associated nosocomial pathogens that accounted for having multiple susceptibility patterns. *Staphylococcus* spp. had fifteen (15) different susceptibility patterns, the most susceptibility patterns of all nosocomial organisms implying that the organisms had fifteen (15) different strains of the same organism making the choice of antibiotic treatment effortless.

92

- *Serratia marcescens* was observed to have five (5) different susceptibility patterns and five (5) different PCR band patterns inferring that five different strains of the same organism existed.

- Infection control practices observed from patient's dockets include chiefly the isolation of MRSA patients and cleaning of infected wounds.

- Four hundred and fifty (450) nosocomial cases were accounted for during the research period from a total of 126,668 admissions at the three (3) regional hospitals with thirty deaths. The nosocomial rate was low 3.6 per 1000 in patients which was good rate when compared to other developing countries.

93

REFERENCES

1) Aliaga L. A clinical index predicting mortality with pseudomonas aeruginosa bacteraemia. *Journal of Medical Microbiology.* 2002; *51(7)*: 615-701.

2) Arbor A.Geriatric oral health and pneumonia risk. *Journal of Clinical Infectious Diseases.* 2005; *40(12):* 1807-1810.

3) Atif ML. Evolution of nosocomial infection prevalence in an algeria university hospital. *Journal of PubMed.* 2006; *36*(8): 423-428.

4) Bjørn B. Surveillance of antimicrobial resistance at a tertiary hospital in tanzania. *BioMed Central Public Health.* 2004; *4*:45.

5) Breathnacha AS. Nosocomial infections. *Journal of Medicine.* 2005; *33*(3): 22-26.

6) Calikoglu S. Hospital pay-for-performance programs in maryland produced strong results, including reduced hospital- acquired conditions. *Health Affairs.* 2012; *31(12):* 2649-2658.

7) Coignard B. National point prevalence survey of healthcare associated infections: results for people aged 65 and older, france. *Journal of the American Geriatrics Society.* 2006; *59(4)*: 763-765.

8) Coopersmith CM. Effect of an education program on decreasing catheter-related bloodstream infections in the surgical intensive care unit. *Crit Care Med.* 2002; *30*(1): 59-64.

9) Crnich CJ.The promise of novel technology for the prevention of intravascular device-related bloodstream infection pathogenesis and short-term devices. *Journal of Clinical Infectious Diseases.* 2002; *34*(9): 1232-1242.

10) David ER. Reducing surgical site infections: a review. *Rev Obstet Gynecol.* 2009; *2*(4): 212-221.

11) Dennis LS. Practice guidelines for the diagnosis and management of skin and soft tissue infections: 2014 update by the infectious diseases society of america. *Clin Infect Dis.* 2015; *59*(2): e10-52.

12) Dia NM. Prevalence of nosocomial infections in a university hospital dakar, senegal. *Med Mal Infect.* 2008; *38*(5): 270-274.

13) DiGiovine B. The attributable mortality and costs of primary nosocomial bloodstream infections in the intensive care unit. *Am J of Respir Crit Care Med.* 1999; *160*(3): 976-981.

94

14) Dixon RE. Nosocomial respiratory infections. *Infect Control*. 1983; *4*(5): 376-381.

15) Ducel G. Prevention of hospital-acquired infections: a practical guide. Geneva, Switzerland: World Health Organization; 2002.

16) Durand ML. Acute bacterial meningitis in adults: a review of 493 episodes. *N Engl J Med*. 1993; *328*(1): 21-28.

17) ECDPC. Annual epidemiological report on communicable diseases in europe. Stockholm, Europe: European Centre for Disease Prevention and Control; 2010.

18) Eggiman P. Impact of a prevention strategy targeted at vascular-access care of incidence of infections acquired in intensive care. *Lancet*. 2000; *355*(9218): 1864-1868.

19) Erik KA. Nosocomial infections. *Internal Medicine*. 2007; *11*(3): 1-16.

20) Ferguson F, Harvey K and Webster K. *Eighteen deaths reported following infections at university of west indies and cornwall regional hospitals*.http://radiojamaicanewsonline.com/local/eighteen-deaths-reported-following-infections-at-uwi-and-cornwall-regional-hospitals [Accessed 20th October 2015].

21) Vrijens F, Hulstaert F, Devriese S and Sande van de S. Hospital- acquired infections in Belgian acute-care hospitals: an estimation of their global impact on mortality, length of stay and health care costs. *Epidemiol Infect*. 2012; *140(1)*: 126-136.

22) Friedman B. Occupational exposure to bloodborne pathogens; needlestick and other sharp injuries; final rule. *OSHA*. 2001; *29(1910)*: H370A.

23) Garner JS. CDC definitions for nosocomial infections. *Am J Infect Control*. 1998; *16*(3): 128-140.

24) Gosling R. Prevalence of hospital-acquired infections in a tertiary referral hospital in northern tanzania. *Ann Trop Med Parasitol*. 2003; *97*(1): 69-73.

25) Grohskpof LS. A national point-prevalence survey of pediatric intensive care unit-acquired infections in the United States. *J Pediatr*. 2002; *140*(4): 432-438.

26) Hugonnet S. Alcohol-based handrub improves compliance with hand hygiene in intensive care units. *Arch Intern Med*. 2002; *162*(9): 1037- 1043.

27) Imam TH. *Bacterial urinary tract infections*. USA: Merck & Co., Inc., Rahway, NJ, USA; 2023.

28) Iyad NM. Incidence rate and distribution of pediatric nosocomial infections. *Pakistan Journal of Pharmacology*. 2007; *24*(1): 53-59.

95

29) Jones JS. (1995). Stethoscopes: A potential vector of infection. *Ann Emerg Med.* 1995; *26*(3): 296-299.

30) Jozsef É. *Italy outraged by horror hospital.* Rome: Liberation Publishing; 2007.

31) Kenrad EN. Infectious disease epidemiology theory and practice. *American Journal of Epidemiology.* 2007; *167*(8): 1014-1015.

32) Klevens RM. (2007). Estimating health care-associated infections and deaths in united states hospitals, 2002. *Public Health Rep.* 2007; *122*(2): 160-166.

33) Laville S. *Jamaica battles hospital infections that have killed 18 babies in three months.*https://www.theguardian.com/world/2015/oct/20/jamaica-hospital-infections-killed-babies [Accessed 20th October 2022].

34) Levy SB. *The antibiotic paradox: how miracle drugs are destroying the miracle.* New York: Plenum Press; 1993.

35) Liu PY. Use of PCR to study epidemiology of serratia marcescens isolates in nosocomial infection. *J Clin Microbiol.* 1994; *32*(8): 1935-1938.

36) Liu C, Purushothama V and Baron S. *Infections of the Respiration System: Medical Micrbiology.* 4th ed.Galveston, TX: University of Texas Medical Branch: 1996.

37) Liziolia A. Prevalence of nosocomial infections in italy: result from the lombardy survey in 2000.*J Hosp Infect.* 2003; *54*(2): 141-148.

38) Lyytikainen O. Antimicrobial use in finnish acute care hospitals: data from national prevalence survey, 2005. *J Antimicrob Chemother Hosp.* 2007; *60*(2): 440-444.

39) Mace SE. Acute bacterial meningitis. *Emergency Medicine Clinics of North America.* 2008; *26*(2): 281-317.

40) Maki DG. Prevention of central venous catheter-related bloodstream infection by use of an antiseptic-impregnated catheter. A randomized, control trial. *Arch Intern Med.* 1997; *127*(4): 257-266.

41) Marinella MA. The stethoscope: a potential source of nosocomial infection.*Arch Intern Med.*1997; *157*(7): 786-790.

42) Martin GS. The epidemiology of sepsis in the united states from 1979 through 2000.*N Engl J Med.* 2003; *348*(16): 1546-1554.

43) Mermel LA. Prevention of intravascular catheter related infections. *Annals Internal Medicine.* 2000; *132*(5): 1-5.

96

44) Moet GJ. Contempory causes of skin and soft tissue infections in north america, latin america and europe: a report from the SENTRY antimicrobial surveillance program (1998-2004). *Diagn Microbiol Infect Dis.*2007; *57*(1): 7-13.

45) Morris A. Nosocomial bacterial meningitis, including central nervous system shunt infections. *InfectDis Clin of North Am.* 1999; *13*(3): 735-750.

46) Muder RR. Pneumonia in residents of long term care facilities: epidemiology, etiology, management and prevention. *Am J Med.* 1998; *105(*4): 319-330.

47) NCCLS. Performance standards for antimicrobial disk susceptibility tests; approved standard. *Clinical and Laboratory Standards Institute.* 2000; *23*(1): M2-A9.

48) NCSL. Hospital-acquired infections: states and public reporting. *Legislative Summit.* Louisville, Washington, DC: National Conference of State Legislatures; 2010.

49) Niederman M. Guidelines for the management of adults with hospital acquired, ventilator associated and healthcare-associated pneumonia. *Am J Respir Crit Care Med.* 2005; *171*(4): 388-416.

50) NNIS. National nosocomial infections surveillance system report; data summary from January 1992 through june 2004.*Am J Infect Control.* 2004; *32*(8): 470-485.

51) Orrett FA. Paediatric nosocomial urinary tract infection at a regional hospital. *International Urology and Nephrology.* 1999; *31*(2): 173-179.

52) Orrett FA. Nosocomial infections in a rural regional hospital in a developing country: infection rates by site, service, cost and infection control practices. *Infect Control Hosp Epidemiol.* 1998; *19*(2): 136-40.

53) Orrett FA. Nosocomial infections in an intensive care unit in a private hospital. *West Indian Medical Journal.* 2000; *51*(1): 21- 24.

54) Pelke S. Gowning does not affect colonization or infection rates in a neonatal intensive care unit. *Archives of Pediatric Adolescence Medicine.* 1994; *148*(10): 1016-1020.

55) Pitt TL. State of the art: typing of serratia marcescens. *J Hosp Infect.* 1982; *3*(1): 9-14.

56) Pittet D. Nosocomial bloodstream infections: secular trends in rates, mortality and contribution to total hospital deaths. *Arch Intern Med.* 1995; *155*(11): 1177-1184.

57) Pollack A. Rising threat of infections unfazed by antibioitics. *New York Times.*2010; *1*(27): 1-29.

97

58) Qiagen. DNeasy Blood and Tissue Handbook, 2006. Austin, TX: Qiagen Group; 2006.

59) Quenon JL. Enquête nationale de prévalence des infections nosocomiales, 1996. *Elsevier.* 1990; *27*(11): 931-934.

60) Raad ID. Central venous catheter coated with minocycline and rifampin for the preventions of catheter-related colonization and bloodstream infection: a randomized, double-blind trial.The texas medical center catheter study group. *Ann Intern Med.* 1997; *127*(4): 267-274.

61) Raimundo GC. (2010). Phenotypic and genotypic characterization of serratia marcescens from a neonatal unit in belém, pará state, brazil. *American Journal Experts.* 2010; *1*(1): 101-106.

62) Merzougui L, Barhoumi T, Guizani T, Barhoumi H, Hannachi H, Turki E, et al. Nosocomial infections in the intensive care unit: annual incidence rate and clinical aspects. *Pan African Medical Journal.* 2018; *30(143)*: 13824.

63) RamakrishnanK.Skin and soft tissue infections. *Am Fam Physician.* 2015; *92*(6): 474-483.

64) RaymondJ. Nosocomial infections in pediatric patients: a european, multicenter prospective study; European study group. *Infect Control Hosp Epidemiol.* 2000; *21*(4): 260-263.

65) Rello J. (2000). Evaluation of outcome of intravenous catheter-related infections in critically ill patients. *Am J Respir Crit Care Med.* 2000; *162*(3): 1027-1030.

66) Richards MJ. (1999). Nosocomial infections in pediatric intensive care units in the united states; national nosocomial infections surveillance system. *Pediatrics.* 1999; *103*(4): e39.

67) Richards MJ. (2000). Nosocomial infections in combined medical surgical intensive care units in the United States. *Infect Control Hosp Epidemiol.* 2000; *21*(8): 510-515.

68) Robert LW. Contamination level of stethoscopes used by physicians and physician assistants. *The Journal of Physician Assistant Education.* 2007; *18*(2): 41-43.

69) Roland N. Penetration of drugs through the blood- cerebrospinal fluid/blood-brain barrier for treatment of central nervous system infections. *Clin Microbiol Rev.* 2010; *23*(4): 858-883.

70) Sherertz RJ. Education of physicians in training can decrease the risk for vascular catheter infection. *Ann Intern Med.* 2000; *132*(8): 641-648.

98

71) Simor A. Molecular and epidemiologic study of multiresistant serratia marcescens infections in a spinal cord Injury rehabilitation unit. *Infect Control Hosp Epidemiol.* 1988; *9*(1): 20-27.

72) Slaughter SA. Comparison of the effect of universal use of gloves and gowns with that of glove use alone on acquisition of vancomycin-resistant enterococci in a medical intensive care unit. *Ann Intern Med.* 1996; *125*(6): 448-456.

73) Smith RL. Excess mortality in critically ill patients with nosocomial bloodstream infections. *Chest.* 1991; *100*(1): 164-167.

74) Soek GT. Does routine gowning reduce nosocomial infection and mortality rates in neonatal nursery? A singapore experience. *Int J of Nurs Pract.* 1995; *1*(1): 52-58.

75) Strausbaugh LJ. Emerging health care-associated infections in the geriatric population. *Emerg Infect Dis.* 2001; *7*(2): 268-271.

76) Théodora AA. Prevalence of nosocomial infections and anti-infective therapy in benin: results of the first nationwide survey in 2012. *Antimicrobial Resistance and Infection Control.* 2014; *3(17),* 1-17.

77) Toni PG. Genotyping of clinical serratia marcescens isolates: a comparision of PCR-based methods. *FEMS Microbiology letters.* 2001; *194(1)*: 19-25.

78) Urrea M. Prospective incidence study of nosocomial infections in a pediatric intensive care unit. *Pediatr Infect Dis J.* 2003; *22*(6): 490-494.

79) Vasselle A. Report on the policy for the fight against nosocomial infections. *Parliamentary Office for the Evaluation of Health Policies.* 2006; *3188*(421): 1-290.

80) Versalovic J. Distribution of repetitive DNA sequences in eubacteria and application to fingerprinting of bacterial genomes. *Nucleic Acids Res.* 1991; *19*(24): 6823-6831.

81) Vincent JL. The prevalence of nosocomial infection in intensive care units in europe: results of the european prevalence of infection in intensive care study. *JAMA.* 1995; 274(8): 639-644.

82) Vincent K. Bacterial skin and soft tissue in adults: a review of their epidemiology, pathogenesis, diagnosis, treatment and site of care. *Can J Infect Dis Med Microbiol.* 2008; *19*(2): 173-184.

83) Vinh DC. Rapidly progressive soft tissue infections. *Lancet Infect Dis.* 2005; *5*(8): 501-513.

99

84) Wayne PA.Performance standards for antimicrobial susceptibility testing. *Clinical and Laboratory Standards Institute*. 2014; *34*(1): M100-S24.

85) WHO,Part 1 Review of Scientific Data Related to Hand Hygiene. WHO Guidelines on Hand Hygiene in Health Care. Geneva, Switzerland: WHO Press; 2009.

86) Yu VL. Serratia marcescens historical perspective a clinical review.*N Engl J Med*. 1979; *300*(16): 887-893.

87) Zelenitsky SA. Treatment and outcome of pseudomonas aeruginosa bacteraemia: an antibiotic pharmacodynamic analysis.*J Antimicrob Chemother*. 2003; *52*(4): 668-674.

88) Wiseman AC. Immunosuppressive Medications. *Clin J Am Soc Nephrol*. 2016; 11(2): 332-343.

100

7.0 APPENDICES

7.1 APPENDIX A

Nosocomial Infections in Trinidad & Tobago

7.1 <u>Questionnaire Form</u>

Patient Code # _____ Sex _____ Age _____

Research Site: (a) EWMSC [ ]   (b) POSGH [ ]   (c) SFG [ ]

Ward _____   Lab # _____

PATIENT HISTORY:

- Is this patient's first visit to hospital?

  (a) Yes [ ]   (b)   No [ ]

- If yes, how long ago was patient admitted to hospital?

  - Year(s) [ ]   (b) month(s) [ ]   (c) week(s) [   ]   (d) day(s) [ ]

- What was the reason for patient's admittance to hospital?

  _____

- Has patient ever had a nosocomial infection?

  - Yes [ ]   (b) no [ ]

- If yes, Frequency of Nosocomial related infection?

  - Once [ ] (b) Twice [ ] (c) Three times [ ] (d) More than four times [ ]

101

- How long ago?

  - A week [ ]   (b) a month [   ] (c) a year [   ] (d) other [   ]

    _____

- Who diagnosed nosocomial infection?

  _____

- How many patients were admitted on ward?

  _____

- Of total number of patients admitted on ward, how many patients had nosocomial infections?

  _____

- Type of Infection

  - (a) SSTI [ ]   (b) GIT [ ]   (c) RT [ ]   (d) UTI [ ]   (e) CNS [ ]
    (f) Blood [ ](g) Other _____

- Mode of spread _____

- What type health service was provided?

  _____

- What was the cost of treating patient with nosocomial infection?

  _____

102

PRESENT HISTORY

Date of admission   ( )   ( )   ( )

          DD   MM   YY

Date of onset ( )   ( )   ( )

                   DD   MM   YY

Was the patient treated with antibiotics in the week(s) prior to admission?

 (a) Yes [ ]   (b) No [ ]

If, yes please state the name of antibiotics

_____

Duration of Hospital Stay (in days)

(a) 2 – 7 days [   ]   (b) 8-14 days [   ] (c) 15 – 21 days [   ] (d) 22 – 28 days (e) >

28 days [   ]

Documented acute complications

(a) Prolong fever [   ]   (b) Seizures [   ]   (c) Subdural emphysema [   ]   (d)

Death [   ]

(e) Other, [   ] please specify   _____

Antibiotic Administered:

- _____ (ii) _____

Did patient have any antibiotic resistance to the antibiotics given?

- Yes [ ]   (b) no [   ]

103

LABORATORY DATA

- **Specimen Source**

(a) Blood [   ]   (b) CSF [   ]   (c) Sputum   [   ]   (d) Pleural fluid   [   ]

(e) Wound swab/Pus   [   ]   (f) Skin & Soft tissue [   ]   (g) Other

_____

- **Other organisms recovered?**

(a) Yes   [   ]   (b) No [   ]

If yes, what organism? _____

- Causative Micro-organisms

  (a) Staphylococcus aureus   [   ]
  (b) Methicillin resistant Staphylococcus aureus   [   ]
  (c) Candida albicans   [   ]
  (d) Pseudomonas aeruginosa   [   ]
  (e) Clostridium difficile   [   ]
  (f) Vancomycin-resistant Enterococcus   [   ]
  (g) Other   _____

- Predisposing Factors (Risk Factors):

  (a) Immuno-compromised patients   [   ]

  (b) Maternal or new-born infections   [   ]

  (c) Chronic diseases:

      (i) Chronic obstructive pulmonary diseases   [   ]

(ii) Chronic Hepatisis C virus   [   ]

(iii) Chronis hemodialysis   [   ]

(iv) Other   _____

- Invasive Devices:

    (i) Catheters   [   ]

    (ii)   Surgical drains   [   ]

    (iii)   Tracheostomy tubes   [   ]

    (iv)   Patients Treatments:

        (a) Immunosuppression   [   ]

        (b) Antacids   [   ]

        (c) Antimicrobial therapy   [   ]

        (d) Blood Transfusion   [   ]

- Treatment Received

    _____

- Outcome

- Cured [ ] (b) transferred to another hospital [ ]   (c) died [ ]   (d) other

    _____

Infection control instituted during patient's management:

_____

105

7.2 APPENDIX B

fair copies   *Ethics Consent*

THE UNIVERSITY OF THE WEST INDIES
ST AUGUSTINE, TRINIDAD AND TOBAGO, WEST INDIES
FACULTY OF MEDICAL SCIENCES
ETHICS COMMITTEE
Telephone: (868) 645-2640 Ext. 5025 Fax: (868) 663-9836 e-mail: deanfms@sta.uwi.edu

May 1, 2012

Dr. Patrick Akpaka
Pathology/Microbiology Unit
Faculty of Medical Sciences
The University of the West Indies
St. Augustine

Dear Dr. Akpaka

Nosocomial infections in Trinidad and Tobago

I am pleased to advise that your application for research on the above captioned topic was approved by Ethics Committee.

Yours sincerely

Shivananda Nayak (Dr.)
Chairman, Ethics Committee
Faculty of Medical Sciences

/erf

106

7.3 APPENDIX C

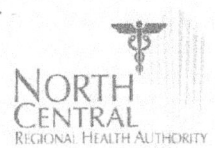

OFFICE OF THE CHIEF EXECUTIVE OFFICER
3rd Floor, Building 39, Eric Williams Medical Sciences Complex, Uriah Butler Highway, Champs Fleurs
PBX: (868)-645-2640   Ext: 2490 / 3089 / 3053   D.L. (868)-662-5579   Fax: (868)-663-0671

October 17, 2012

Ms. Camille Elliott
MPhil Student
Department of Para-Clinical Sciences
Faculty of Medical Sciences
The University of the West Indies
EWMSC

Dear Ms. Elliott,

Approval to Conduct Research Project in the NCRHA

Reference is made to the subject at caption.

Please be informed that approval has been granted for research entitled – *"Nosocomial Infections in Trinidad and Tobago"*.

The NCRHA wishes you every success in this undertaking, and looks forward to receiving a copy of your Project Report in the near future.

Sincerely,

Mr. Collin Bissessar
Chief Executive Officer (Ag)

x.c: Mr. Ashford Sankar – Chief Operations Officer, NCRHA
       Mr. Kawal Singh – Human Resources Consultant
       Public Health Observatory, NCRHA

107

7.4 APPENDIX D

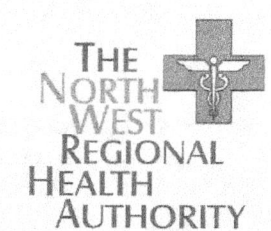

Office of the General Manager,
Health Policy Research and Planning

North West Regional Health Authority
#39 Dundonald Street
Port of Spain
Tel: 625-1295 ext. 215, 245
Fax 623-3310
Email: health.services@nwrha.co.tt

November 15th, 2012

Ms Camille Elliot
Student
Para Clinical Science
University of the West Indies
St Augustine

Dear Ms. Elliot

Re: Nosocomial Infection in Trinidad and Tobago

The North West Regional Health Authority (NWRHA) wishes to convey approval to conduct the aforementioned study.

Please be advised that all findings are to be submitted to the office of the **Chief Executive Officer, North West Regional Health Authority, #39 Dundonald Street, Port-of-Spain** upon completion of research and before publication of same.

Thank you for your co-operation.

Yours sincerely

Mrs. Lauren K. Maharaj
General Manager,
Health Policy Research and Planning
NWRHA
Secretary, Ethics Committee

108

7.5 APPENDIX E

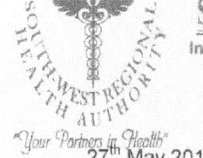

SOUTH-WEST REGIONAL HEALTH AUTHORITY

Independence Avenue, Paradise Pasture, San Fernando, Trinidad & Tobago, West Indies.
Phone: PBX (868) 653-4259 / 9096 / 0724 / 8078, 652-6810, 657-9872
Fax: PBX ext 2301
Email: info@swrha.co.tt   Website: www.swrha.co.tt

"Your Partners in Health"
27th May 2013

Ms. Camille Elliot
c/o Dr. Patrick E Akpaka
BMQ Building
San Fernando General Hospital

Dear Ms. Elliot

Re: Approval of Research Project

Please be advised that permission has been given to you to conduct your research project entitled *"Nosocomial infections in Trinidad and Tobago."*

The South-West Regional Health Authority thanks you for selecting San Fernando General Hospital to conduct your research. However, it is important to note that this Region has a **confidentiality policy**.

Also note, that approval must be sought from the Clinical Governance and Ethics Committee, South West Regional Health Authority before data collected can be published or presented in any way outside of your university assignment.

At the completion of the research project, **a final report must** be submitted to the Clinical Governance and Ethics Committee for our records within six (6) months of completion.

The Authority wishes you the very best in your future endeavours.

Sincerely

Dr. Shevanand Gopeesingh
Chairman, Clinical Governance & Ethics Committee

c   Dr. Anand Chatoorgoon,   Medical Director
      Mr. Praimlal Ramcharan,   Hospital Administrator Ag.

www.ingramcontent.com/pod-product-compliance
Lightning Source LLC
Chambersburg PA
CBHW081425220526
45466CB00008B/2274